THE DEAD MO

The Dead Mother brings together original essays in honour of André Green. Written by distinguished psychoanalysts, the collection develops the theme of his most famous paper of the same title, and describes the value of relating the concept of the dead mother to other areas of clinical interest: psychic reality, borderline phenomena, passions, identification.

The concept of the 'dead mother' describes a clinical phenomenon, sometimes difficult to identify, but always present in a substantial number of patients. It describes a process by which the image of a living and loving mother is transformed into a distant figure; a toneless, practically inanimate, dead parent. In reality, the mother remains alive, but she has psychically 'died' for the child. This produces a depression in the child, who carries these feelings within him or her into adult life, as the experience of the loss of the mother's love is followed by the loss of meaning in life. Nothing makes sense any more for the child, but life seems to continue under the appearance of normality.

The Dead Mother is a valuable contribution to literature on psychoanalytic and psychotherapeutic approaches to grief, loss and depression.

Gregorio Kohon is a Training Analyst from the British Psycho-Analytical Society. He works in private practice in London. Contributors: Martin S. Bergmann; Christopher Bollas; André Green; André Lussier; Arnold H. Modell; Thomas H. Ogden; Michael Parsons; Rosine Jozef Perelberg; Adam Phillips; Jed Sekoff.

THE NEW LIBRARY OF PSYCHOANALYSIS
General Editor Dana Birksted-Breen

The New Library of Psychoanalysis was launched in 1987 in association with the Institute of Psychoanalysis, London. It took over from the International Psychoanalytical Library which published many of the early translations of the works of Freud and the writings of most of the leading British and Continental psychoanalysts.

The purpose of the New Library of Psychoanalysis is to facilitate a greater and more widespread appreciation of psychoanalysis and to provide a forum for increasing mutual understanding between psychoanalysts and those working in other disciplines such as the social sciences, medicine, philosophy, history, linguistics, literature and the arts. It aims to represent different trends both in British psychoanalysis and in psychoanalysis generally. The New Library of Psychoanalysis is well placed to make available to the English-speaking world psychoanalytic writings from other European countries and to increase the interchange of ideas between British and American psychoanalysts.

The Institute, together with the British Psychoanalytical Society, runs a low-fee psychoanalytic clinic, organizes lectures and scientific events concerned with psychoanalysis and publishes the *International Journal of Psychoanalysis*. It also runs the only UK training course in psychoanalysis which leads to membership of the International Psychoanalytical Association – the body which preserves internationally agreed standards of training, of professional entry, and of professional ethics and practice for psychoanalysis as initiated and developed by Sigmund Freud. Distinguished members of the Institute have included Michael Balint, Wilfred Bion, Ronald Fairbairn, Anna Freud, Ernest Jones, Melanie Klein, John Rickman and Donald Winnicott.

Previous General Editors include David Tuckett, Elizabeth Spillius and Susan Budd. Previous and current Members of the Advisory Board include Christopher Bollas, Ronald Britton, Catalina Bronstein, Donald Campbell, Sara Flanders, Stephen Grosz, John Keene, Eglé Laufer, Juliet Mitchell, Michael Parsons, Rosine Jozef Perelberg, Richard Rusbridger, David Taylor and Mary Target.

ALSO IN THIS SERIES

TITLES IN THE NEW LIBRARY OF
PSYCHOANALYSIS TEACHING SERIES

THE DEAD MOTHER

The Work of André Green

Edited by Gregorio Kohon

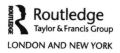

Routledge
Taylor & Francis Group

LONDON AND NEW YORK

First published 1999
by Routledge
27 Church Road, Hove, East Sussex BN3 2FA

Simultaneously published in the USA and Canada
by Routledge
711 Third Avenue, New York, NY 10017 (8th Floor)

Routledge is an imprint of the Taylor & Francis Group, an Informa business

Typeset in Bembo by Routledge

British Library Cataloguing in Publication Data
A catalogue record for this book is available from the British Library

Library of Congress Cataloguing in Publication Data
The dead mother: the work of André Green/[edited by]
Gregorio Kohon. Includes bibliographical references and index.
1. Psychoanalysis. 2. Grief. 3. Loss (Psychology). 4. Depression,
Mental. 5. Green, André. I. Kohon, Gregorio. II. Series.
BF175.D387 1999   99–12420
150.19´5´092–dc21   CIP

ISBN 978–0–415–16529–7 (pbk)

CONTENTS

CONTENTS

CONTRIBUTORS

Martin S. Bergmann is Clinical Professor of Psychology at the New York University Post-Doctoral Program. He is Training and Supervising psychoanalyst at the New York Freudian Society, and an honorary member of the American Psychoanalytic Association. He is the author of *The Anatomy of Loving: A Man's Quest to Know What Love is* and *In the Shadow of Moloch: The Sacrifice of Children and Its Impact on Western Religions*. He co-authored *Generations of the Holocaust* and *The Evolution of Psychoanalytic Technique*. His book, *An Evaluation of the Hartmann Era*, the proceedings of a conference in which André Green played a major role, was published by The Other Press (1999).

Christopher Bollas is a psychoanalyst in private practice in London. He has published, among other books, *Cracking Up – The Work of Unconscious Experience*, and *The New Informants – Betrayal of Confidentiality in Psychoanalysis and Psychotherapy* (with David Sundelson). His next book to be published is *The Mystery of Things*.

Gregorio Kohon is a Training analyst, British Psycho-Analytical Society. In 1988, he co-founded with Valli Shaio Kohon the Brisbane Centre for Psychoanalytic Studies, which he directed until December 1994. He is the editor of *The British School of Psychoanalysis – The Independent Tradition* (London: Free Association Books, 1986). His book *No Lost Certainties to be Recovered* (1999) was published by Karnac. He works in private practice.

André Lussier was Full Professor of Psychoanalysis, at the University of Montreal (1953–1986); past Vice-President of the International Psychoanalytic Association; past President, Canadian Psychoanalytic Society; past President, Société Psychanalytique de Montréal; past Director, Canadian Psychoanalytic Institute.

Arnold H. Modell is Clinical Professor of Psychiatry, Harvard Medical School, and a Training and Supervising analyst, Boston Psychoanalytic Institute. He is the author of *Other Times, Other Realities* and *The Private Self*.

Thomas H. Ogden, MD, is Co-Director of the Center for the Advanced Study of the Psychoses. He is a member of the editorial board for North America of *The International Journal of Psycho-Analysis*, and the author of five books on the theory and practice of psychoanalysis. His most recent publications are *Reverie and Interpretation*; *Sensing Something Human*; and *Subjects of Analysis*. He supervises, teaches and conducts a private practice of psychoanalysis in San Francisco.

Michael Parsons is a Training Analyst, British Psycho-Analytical Society. He co-edited *Before I was I – Psychoanalysis and the Imagination*, a collection of papers by Enid Balint. His book *The Dove that Returns, The Dove that Vanishes* is forthcoming.

Rosine Jozef Perelberg PhD is a Training Analyst, British Psycho-Analytical Society. She gained her PhD in Social Anthropology at the London School of Economics, London. She has edited *Gender and Power in Families* (co-edited with Anne Miller, 1990); *Female Experience: Three Generations of British Women Psychoanalysts on Work With Women* (co-edited with Joan Raphael-Leff, 1997); and *Psychoanalytic Understanding of Violence and Suicide*, 1998. For the last ten years she has been working at The Anna Freud Centre on a research project which offers subsidised analysis to young adults. She is also in private practice.

Adam Phillips is a child psychotherapist working in London. His most recent publication is *The Beast in the Nursery*. His next book is entitled *Darwin's Worms*. He is the editor of the new Penguin Freud.

Jed Sekoff is a psychoanalyst practising in Berkeley, California.

PREFACE

Gregorio Kohon's idea – a collection of essays in honour of André Green's 70th birthday – is no doubt an act of justice, and one with particular value for psychoanalysis. André Green is one of the most distinguished analysts of our time. His work encompasses a body of theory of singular importance that has permeated psychoanalytic thinking in France, all of Europe, and Latin America. In the English-speaking psychoanalytic community, Green is known mostly through his presentations at international congresses, professional visits, and through personal contacts; but little of his writing has found its way into English. This is in sharp contrast to the Spanish-speaking world. In Argentina, for example, there are study groups in Buenos Aires led by Reggy Serebriany, Manuel Galvez, and other distinguished psychoanalysts, where Green's work is taught and discussed.

Aged 19, André Green arrived in Paris in 1946. He decided to study medicine, with the expressed purpose of devoting himself to psychiatry. This vocation had emerged from a long way back, and as soon as he qualified as a doctor he began his psychiatric training in 1953. This was a very special moment, when the psychotropic era begun. At the same time, a major upheaval shook the Société Psychoanalytique de Paris, when Lagache, Lacan and other important members broke away to form the Association Psychana-lytique de France.

After winning a position at the famed St Anne's Hospital, where he worked with Henry Ey, Green entered psychoanalysis, following the advice of one of his outstanding teachers (Julián de Aguariaguerra). His first analyst was Maurice Bouvet, from 1956 until his premature death in 1960. After this initial experience, valuable but unfinished, Green completed his analysis with Jean Mallet and afterwards with Catherine Parat.

After the Bonneval Colloquium in 1960, Green decide to attend Lacan's seminar, while keeping his affiliation to the Société Psychanalytique de Paris. At the same time, he had the chance of meeting the most prominent members of the British Psycho-Analytical Society. Through difficult and passionate years of intense psychoanalytic debates and disagreements, Green managed to keep a somewhat fluid balance between different groups and personalities. This was a sure sign of his independent mind. Nevertheless, this balance was first shaken by the publication of *Le Narcissisme primaire: structure ou état*, written in 1966 and published two years later. There Green argued that primary narcissism could only be understood as a structure. After endorsing Freud's notions of the existence of defences prior to repression (turning against the self and reversal into the opposite – which Green calls 'double inversion'), he concluded his book suggesting that primary narcissism is the Desire of One under the trace of the Other, the subject's aspiration for a self-sufficient and immortal totality.

The final break away from Lacan came about as a result of his Report to the Congrès de Psychanalystes de Langues Romanes in 1970, where he criticised Lacan's theory of the signifier, bringing into question the notion of the unconscious structured as a language. Three years later, this Report became a book, *Le Discours vivant*, establishing Green as a prestigious author.

In 1973, Green wrote (together with J. L. Donnet) a seminal book, *L'Enfant de Ça*, where he introduced the concept of *psychose blanche*. Some of his findings were summarised and presented in the paper read at the 29th International Psycho-Analytical Congress (London, 1975), 'The analyst, symbolization and absence in the analytic setting', which constituted an important moment in Green's theoretical development. Green suggested a new dual conception of anxiety, separation anxiety and intrusion anxiety, connected not to the question of the wish (as in neurosis), but to the development of thought. The triangular Oedipal situation is antedated in his theoretical formulation by an earlier 'bi-triangulation', where the relationship takes place between the subject and two symmetrically opposed objects (which disguises the splitting of a single object – the two are in fact one entity). From this point onward, Green deepens his research on the work of the negative and the concept of blank psychosis.

This is not the place to trace the complex itinerary of André Green's prolific work. His theoretical contributions are many and very important, as are his books and papers on applied psychoanalysis in regard to Greek tragedy, Shakespearean drama, or the work of Proust, Sartre, Borges, and others. Green is a Freudian analyst who has managed to integrate in a lucid synthesis the influence of authors as diverse as Lacan, Bion, and, especially, Winnicott. He believes that psychoanalysis should find its own theories and develop its own forms of research. In this context, he has strongly opposed empirical investigation and baby observation, two methods that he sees as alien to psychoanalysis.

Kohon has selected a remarkable array of psychoanalysts to contribute to this book, some of whom are very famous authors in their own right. The title of the collection, *The Dead Mother*, refers to one of Green's fundamental contributions. The concept of the dead mother describes a clinical phenomenon, sometimes difficult to identify, but always present in certain patients: the subject, as a child, has suddenly (unconsciously) realised that his or her mother has become depressed and things are not the same as before; she is there, but now she feels dead, absent. The depression of the mother might produce a blank mourning, which does not result from the interplay of the mechanisms of introjection and projection, but from a process of decathexis, of disinvestment (in accordance with Winnicott's subjective object).

The concept of the dead mother is a structural concept – even though it is found in the concrete experience of the subject's childhood. While in Lacan's theory there is the concept of the dead father, which represents the continuity of the previous generations through the superego (the Law of the father), the concept of the dead mother (although not a transgenerational phenomenon) comes to re-establish a balance between the two parental figures in psychoanalytic theory. The whole of Green's theoretical endeavour could be described as the articulation of primary narcissism with the death instinct, through his concept of negative narcissism.

I wish to end on a personal note. When André Green visited Argentina for the first time in 1974, I listened to his presentations with enormous interest. My wife invited André to our home, and thus began a friendship which has endured for over a quarter of a century.

R. Horacio Etchegoyen
Past President,
The International Psychoanalytic Association,
January 1999

ACKNOWLEDGEMENTS

Most of the papers included in this collection were written by their authors especially for this book. There are three exceptions: André Green's 'The intuition of the negative in *Playing and Reality*', published in *the International Journal of Psycho-Analysis*, 1997, Vol. 78, Part 6, pp 1071–1084, and Thomas H. Ogden's 'Analysing forms of aliveness and deadness of the transference–countertransference', published in *The International Journal of Psycho-Analysis*, 1995, Vol. 76, Part 4, pp. 695–709. Parts of Rosine Perelberg's 'The interplay of identifications: violence, hysteria and the repudiation of femininity' have been published in *The International Journal of Psycho-Analysis*, 1999, Vol. 80, Part 1, pp. 31-45. I am grateful to David Tuckett, the editor of the Journal, for his kind permission to reproduce the papers here. I am indebted to Elizabeth Bott Spillius, for her prompt and enthusiastic response to the suggestion for the book. Peter Shaio has been, as usual, very efficient and highly competent in helping me with the original editing of the manuscript. Linda Mason's secretarial skills were an invaluable help. Special thanks to Jill Duncan, Assistant Librarian, The Institute of Psycho-Analysis.

I discovered André Green's writings for the first time in 1969, as a student, just before qualifying as a clinical psychologist. I have followed the development of his ideas since then. I met André Green for the first time in 1993, in Australia, on the occasion of the third international conference hosted by the Brisbane Centre for Psychoanalytic Studies, on Psychoanalysis, Madness and the Theatre. Green opened the conference with an inaugural lecture on Psychoanalysis and Culture, and presented one of the main papers, 'Scenes of tragic madness in Ancient Greece'. It was a memorable occasion, both personal and professional. André Green showed great magnanimity in helping my wife, Valli, and me, to establish a psychoanalytic oasis in Queensland.

Editing this book has been hard work but part of the pleasure in carrying out this project has been the time we spent at the Greens' house in the Luberon, France, in December 1997, when I had the opportunity to interview him over several evenings. My thanks to Litza and André Green for their generous hospitality. An edited version of the eight hours of taped conversation is included as Chapter 1 in this volume. I owe the title for the interview to Lisa Appignanesi.

My deepest gratitude is for the authors who have contributed so generously to the book. Above all, they have been most gracious and patient in responding to my editorial suggestions and demands.

INTRODUCTION

Gregorio Kohon

In 1997, André Green was 70 years old. The idea for the present volume emerged then from a wish to celebrate, in the Anglo-Saxon world, Green's many and varied contributions to psychoanalyis. Green's published psycho-analytic work started with a short paper on 'L'œuvre de Maurice Bouvet' (Green, 1960). Two years later, Green published 'L'inconscient freudien et la psychoanalyse française contemporaine' (Green, 1962). This paper had been delivered as part of a critical exchange with Laplanche and Leclaire, at the Bonneval Colloquium organised by Henry Ey in 1960, on L'Inconscient (Ey, 1966) – where Green also presented a major paper (1966). In that article, Green questioned the validity of the Lacanian formula that the unconscious is structured like a language; he criticised Laplanche and Leclaire for leaving aside some important aspects of the Freudian *Vorstellungs-Repräsentanz*, and for their ignoring the question of affects in their contribution to the Colloquium. Green argued for the need to give priority to the drives in psychoanalysis, and, notably, for the consideration of the subject's conflict between positivity and negativity. He would develop many of these themes later in his work. Towards the end of the paper, he declared that his criticisms did not necessarily separate him from Laplanche and Leclaire; it was more an invitation for a dialogue.

It is this kind of dialogue, with a critical, formidable interlocutor like Green, that the English-speaking reader has been deprived of for many years. Green has written fourteen books and around two hundred articles. He has been translated into many languages, but only two books have been published in English: *The Tragic Effect* (1979), and the collection of papers gathered under the title *On Private Madness* (1986). (In fact, *Le Discours vivant – La conception psychanalytique de l'affect* (1973) will appear in the New Library collection – twenty-six years after its original publication!)

Green's paper on 'The dead mother', which gives its title to the present volume, is undoubtedly his best known work. Originally, it constituted a chapter in his book *Narcissime de vie, narcissisme de mort*, published in 1983; and it was later included in *On Private Madness*. I will offer here a brief summary, using mainly Green's own words.

1

Green argues that what distinguishes present-day analyses is 'the problems of mourning' (1983, p. 142), but he is not going to be talking about the 'real death of the mother'. The dead mother is a concept that refers to:

> an imago which has been constituted in the child's mind, following maternal depression, brutally transforming a living object, which was a source of vitality for the child, into a distant figure, toneless, practically inanimate, deeply impregnating the cathexes of certain patients ... and weighing on the destiny of their object-libidinal and narcissistic future ... [The] dead mother ... is a mother who remains alive but who is, so to speak, psychically dead in the eyes of the young child in her care.
>
> (ibid., p. 142)

Green shares with other authors two central ideas, which form the basis of his theoretical grounding:

> The first is that of *object-loss* as a fundamental moment in the structuring of the human psyche ... The second ... idea is that of a *depressive position* ... a general situation referring to an unavoidable event in the process of development.
>
> (ibid., p.143)

While psychoanalytic theory, according to Green, has given great importance to the dead father, thus emphasising the role of castration and the structuring of the superego, 'we never hear of the dead mother from a structural point of view' (ibid., p. 144). Green gives special importance to this 'structural function', 'a constitutive conception of the psychical order ... programmed by the primal fantasies' (ibid., p. 145). But Green, at this point, dissociates himself from a structural point of view focused on one paradigm, and proposes instead 'at least two' models: one, centred on castration anxiety, '[which] is always evoked in the context of a bodily wound associated with a bloody act' (ibid., p. 145); the other is centred on the anxiety related to all forms of object-loss – which could include, for example, being abandoned by one's own superego. Most importantly, this anxiety 'bears the colours of mourning: black or white. Black as in severe depression, or blank as in states of emptiness' (ibid., p. 146). Green declares:

> I defend the hypothesis that the sinister black of depression, which we can legitimately relate to the hatred we observe in the psychoanalysis of depressed subjects, is only a secondary product, a consequence rather than a cause, of a 'blank' anxiety which expresses a loss that has been experienced on a narcissistic level.
>
> (ibid., p. 146)

2

'Blankness' is a category that has formed part of a series of concepts created by Green: negative hallucination, blank psychosis, blank mourning, all of which are connected to 'the problem of emptiness, or of the negative, in our clinical practice' (ibid., p. 146). For him, 'blankness' is 'the result of one of the components of primary repression: massive decathexis of the maternal primary object, which leaves traces in the unconscious in the form of "psychic holes" ' (ibid., p. 146). But, always Freudian, Green makes it clear that:

> The Oedipus complex should be maintained as the essential symbolic matrix ... However advanced the analysis [of this decathexis] may be, the fate of the human psyche is to have always *two* objects and never one alone, however far one goes back to try to understand the earliest psychical structure.
>
> (ibid., p.146)

Decathexis of the object, psychic holes, blank anxiety, depressive emptiness, the dialectics of presence and absence: '*The essential characteristic of this depression is that it takes place in the presence of the object, which is itself absorbed by a bereavement.* The mother, for one reason or another, is depressed' (ibid., p. 149). The loss could be that of a close person to the mother, or it could originate 'by a deception which inflicts a narcissistic wound'. The important aspect is that, 'In any event the mother's sorrow and lessening of interest in her infant are in the foreground' (ibid., p. 149). Love is suddenly lost for the child; there is a transformation in the infant's world which produces a psychical catastrophe: loss of love is followed by loss of meaning; for the child, nothing makes sense any more. Since 'more often than not' a distant mother is accompanied by an absent father (who refuses, or does not know how to respond to the child); the infant cannot turn to anybody, and is caught in 'a unique movement with two aspects': following the decathexis of the maternal object, the child unconsciously identifies with the mother (ibid., pp.150–1).

The decathexis is an act of 'murder', but the primary object is killed 'without hatred' (ibid., p.151); instead of an object that has been destroyed, there is a psychic hole. Above all, '*the quest for lost meaning structures the early development of the fantasmatic and the intellectual capacities of the ego*' (ibid., p. 152). Nevertheless, the infant needs to survive a life without meaning (one way or another), and for that he/she might develop a *compulsion to imagine* (a frantic need for play), and/or a *compulsion to think* (which promotes intellectual development). There is a hole in the child's psychic world, but this might be covered by a 'patched breast' (ibid., p. 152). In this case, sublimation does not fail after all. We are faced with a paradox: artistic creativity and productive intellectualisation are possible outcomes for the dead mother complex. But this cannot be accomplished without a price being paid: the subject will remain 'vulnerable on a particular point, which is his love life' (ibid., p. 153).

It is in this second instance, in the subject's incapacity for love, where the identification with the dead mother appears more clearly:

> The subject's trajectory evokes a hunt in quest of an introjectable object, without the possibility of renouncing it or losing it, and indeed, the possibility of accepting its introjection into the ego, which is cathected by the dead mother. In all, the subject's objects remain constantly at the limit of the ego, not wholly within, and not quite without. And with good reason, for the place is occupied, in its centre, by the dead mother.
>
> (ibid., pp. 153–4)

> The object has been encapsulated and its trace has been lost through decathexis; primary identification with the dead mother took place, transforming positive identification into negative identification, i.e. identification with the hole left by the decathexis (and not identification with the object), and to this emptiness, which is filled in and suddenly manifests itself through an affective hallucination of the dead mother, as soon as a new object is periodically chosen to occupy this space.
>
> (ibid., p. 155)

Love, then, is not possible, only love which has been frozen by the decathexis, a form of love which keeps the object in hibernation: the subject's love is 'mortgaged to the dead mother'. Autonomy, of a kind. Impossibility of sharing. Solitude, actively sought because it gives the subject the illusion that the dead mother has left him/her alone. Passions, for sure, are not to be experienced; pleasure is not be had. There is, in all cases – says Green – a regression to anality, and (no surprises here) the use of reality as a defence: 'Fantasy must be only fantasy' (ibid., p. 158).

What are the clinical consequences of such a predicament? Green describes them thus: 'The patient is strongly attached to the analysis – the analysis more than the analyst'. The analyst is still a transferential object, but the transference takes 'deep root in a tonality of a narcissistic nature'. The lack of transferential passion is justified by the appeal to 'reality'; if there is any hint of seduction, this takes place in 'the area of the intellectual quest'. And yet, after all is said and done, perhaps not unexpectedly, one can discover something else in the transference: 'behind the dead mother complex, behind the blank mourning for the mother, one catches a glimpse of the mad passion of which she is, and remains, the object, that renders mourning for her an impossible experience' (ibid., p.162).

4

What can be done? The analyst has two choices: if one follows the 'classic solution', then 'the analysis may sink into funereal boredom'. Understandably, Green prefers the second, alternative approach:

> by using the setting as a transitional space, [this approach] makes an ever-living object of the analyst, who is interested, awakened by the analysand, giving proof of his vitality by the associative links he communicates to him, without leaving his neutrality.
>
> (ibid., p. 163)

Not an easy task, and a challenging encounter: an analyst on the side of life versus the 'keeper of the tomb'.

To elaborate on the rich texture of André Green's paper, on the clinical resonances of his discoveries, one would have to place the dead mother complex within the much wider context of Green's other theoretical contributions: the role of the affects; his understanding of object relationships; the importance given by Green to representation, and to the Freudian distinction between thing-representation and word-representation; his insistence on the concept of primary narcissism; his conviction about the theoretical and clinical need for the inclusion of the drives in psychoanalysis, and of cathexis and decathexis; his theory of language; his theory of thinking (not only understood as emerging from the absence of the object but also as the product of a negative hallucination of the maternal object); the concept of blank psychosis, developed in collaboration with Donnet (Donnet and Green, 1973); binding and unbinding; and many more of his contributions.

André Green is a French analyst. This means that he not only belongs to a particular psychoanalytic tradition but to French culture and, more pertinently, French philosophy. Green's work, like that of many other colleagues from France, takes place in the context of an implicit and explicit critical dialogue with Hegel; neo-Kantianism; the inheritance of Bergson, Heidegger, and Husserl; Sartre and Merleau-Ponty; the course given at the Ecole Pratique des Hautes Etudes by Alexandre Kojève (who seemed to have influenced just about everything that has been produced in France after 1940); semiotics; structuralism; Lacan, Foucault and Althusser. Some of the crucial themes discussed in philosophy re-appeared in the theoretical work of the French clinicians: absence; negation, negativity, and nothingness; identity and difference; enunciation and language; perception and truth.

At the same time, while our French colleagues seem to have found the time and the space to study the British contributions to psychoanalysis (offering their own version of Melanie Klein, Bion, Winnicott, Balint, and Fairbairn), most British psychoanalysts have tended to ignore the contributions from across the Channel.

The papers included in this book do not exclusively refer to the concept of the dead mother. The purpose of the collection is, as stated above, to celebrate the contributions of André Green to psychoanalysis. The hope is to make the reader … curious.

Michael Parsons takes negation as 'an essential element in all psychic work, particularly psychoanalytic work'. Furthermore, following Freud's distinction between psychical (internal reality) and external (ordinary) reality, Parsons argues that psychical reality 'is not only a refuge from ordinary reality. The opposite way may also be true.' And he adds, 'If psychic reality is constituted by representation, and representation depends on an act of negation, that makes negation an essential element in the constitution of psychic reality.' In fact, 'the analytic setting is an external representation of the negating which is essential to the creation of psychic reality'. This is related to André Green's work of the negative. According to Parsons, the destructuring use of negation is exemplified in Green's concept of the dead mother.

Arnold Modell is interested in the epistemology of trauma, the question of memory, and the problems of reconstruction in psychoanalysis. He suggests using the concept of the dead mother 'as a paradigm of the child's response to a traumatic disruption'. He makes a distinction between the *dead mother syndrome* and the *dead mother complex*. The syndrome is a malignant clinical presentation, where there is 'a primary identification with the emotionally dead mother', the result of an 'absence of a prolonged affective interaction'. The complex can comprehend an entire range of different responses to a depressed or absent mother.

Christopher Bollas presents the case of Antonio, a man in his thirties who suddenly uses mimicry in one session to take bizarre possession of the analyst, as an attempt to convey an experience with no meaning. Antonio is paranoid, in profound despair, partly psychically crippled, invaded by violent phantasies and peculiar thoughts, and is compelled to turn things in his life sour. Caught in repetition, Antonio can only experience love 'in the maternal necropolis' of the dead mother complex. Instead of love for the object, Antonio wishes 'to nourish the dead mother, to maintain her perpetually embalmed' (Green, 1986, p. 162).

Jed Sekoff is initially inspired by looking at photographs. He states that 'a photograph captures an instant of time, a frozen moment that offers the possibility of holding time in our hands'. In a photograph, 'A dead face lives on'; 'The dead are somehow conjured into life' from a negative. A number of clinical examples allows Sekoff to elaborate on what he calls 'the palette of Green's epistemology of the negative': not only the description of a certain pathological organisation named as the dead mother, but a whole 'project of theorising absence as a fundamental property of psychical life'. Like Bion and Winnicott, Green is said to join them 'as the explorers par excellence' of what might be called the *negative sublime*.

Thomas Ogden explores the analyst's uses of his countertransference experience:

to address specific expressive and defensive roles of the sense of aliveness and deadness of the analysis as well as the particular function of these qualities of experience in the landscape of the patient's internal object world and object relationships.

In the dead mother complex, the issues of deadness and aliveness are crucial. Ogden believes that 'every form of psychopathology represents a specific type of limitation of the individual's capacity to be fully alive as a human being'; therefore the experience of aliveness 'must be considered as an aspect of the analytic experience *in its own terms*', well beyond the commonly accepted goals of the analytic treatment.

André Lussier declares that André Green's concept of the dead mother has become for him 'an indispensable source of inspiration for any work dealing with related clinical psychoanalysis'. Lussier describes how the analysis of a certain number of patients who suffered from the dead mother complex necessarily proceeds 'from the most superficial layers to the very deep'. He centres his meditation on the unconscious identification of the subject with his/her love-object, an identification that aims at avoiding the greater threat of its loss.

Adam Phillips states that:

> Our passionate selves are our best selves; and a passionate life is only possible ... if we can make our passion known: to ourselves, by the absence of the object stimulating desire and its correlative representations, and to the object, through the articulation of love as demand. There can be no passion ... without representation.

Green is one analyst who 'has been able to go on asking the Freudian question: what, if anything, has our passion got to do with so-called other people?' Can representation be the enemy of passion? And yet, without passion, 'the human subject would seem disembodied'; representation is not all. While passion has always been part of psychoanalytic theory, right from the beginning of psychoanalysis, there has also been a wish to push passion out of the picture.

Rosine Jozef Perelberg suggests that Green's concept of the dead mother could be considered a 'core complex' in borderline states. Taking André Green's ideas on the negative as a reference point, Perelberg explores the way in which Green's theoretical notions have helped her to understand two different types of psychopathological phenomena. She suggests that 'what lies at the basis of violence (in certain patients) and hysteria is the repudiation of femininity'. Perelberg presents the case of a violent male patient in analysis and also discusses the case of Anna O.

Martin S. Bergmann believes that some psychoanalytic debates have changed the history of psychoanalysis. Among them, he includes the debate that took place between Leon Rangell and André Green at the London Psychoanalytic Congress of 1975. André Green suggested a 'new theoretical-clinical model ... based on work with borderline patients'. These patients 'aspire to attain a state of emptiness and non-being'. Decathexis is an alternative to repression: 'what has been repressed remains alive'. In the context of these contributions, Green will then proceed to describe the dead mother complex a few years later. By then the concept of decathexis had become central to Green's theoretical work.

André Green makes a parallel between his ideas concerning *the work of the negative* and some of Winnicott's concepts. For example, the 'not-me' possession, in which the object is defined as 'a negative of me'; or the paradox involved in the use of a transitional object, which 'includes a tolerance of the negative'; or the progressive decathexis of an object, which Green characterises as 'a representation of the absence of representation'. The author sees many examples of the negative in Winnicott, and Green believes that he was

> close to a notion that he never had a chance to promote to a theoretical status ... This all refers to a lack: absence of memory, absence in the mind, absence of contact, absence of feeling alive – all these absences can be condensed in the idea of a gap. But that gap, instead of referring to a simple void or to something which is missing, becomes the substratum of what is real.

Green further connects his concepts of the dead mother and of negative hallucination, as well as that of an introjected construction of a framing structure and the disobjectalising function, with Winnicott's own ideas, through the discussion of some clinical material concerning a patient first treated by Winnicott, and later – coincidentally – treated by Green.

References

Donnet, J. L. and Green, A. (1973) *L'enfant de ça. La psychose blanche*. Paris: Editions de Minuit.

Ey, H. (ed.) (1966) *L'Inconscient*. Paris: Desclée de Brouwer.

Green, A. (1960) L'œuvre de Maurice Bouvet. *Revue française de psychanalyse* 24, 1, pp. 685–702.

—— (1962) L'Inconscient freudien et la psychanalyse française contemporaine. *Les Temps Modernes* 195, pp. 365–79.

—— (1966) L'Inconscient et la psychopathologie. *L'Inconscient*, VI Colloque de Bonneval, Paris: Desclée de Brouwer.

—— (1969) *The Tragic Effect: The Oedipus Complex in Tragedy*. Cambridge: Cambridge University Press, 1979.

—— (1973) *Le discours vivant. La conception psychanalytique de l'affect*. Paris: Presses Universitaires de France.

—— (1980) *Narcissisme de vie, narcissisme de mort*. Paris: Editions de Minuit.

—— (1983) The dead mother. In A. Green, *On Private Madness*. London: the Hogarth Press and the Institute of Psychoanalysis, 1986. Original publication, La mère morte. In *Narcissisme de vie, narcissisme de mort*. Paris: Editions de Minuit, pp.222–53.

1

THE GREENING OF PSYCHOANALYSIS

André Green in dialogues with Gregorio Kohon

GK   I actually haven't prepared any specific questions ...

AG   Neither did I.

GK   ... but one thing I thought of asking you is to talk about your life, before we talk about your work.

AG   As you may know, there are two books that have been written about me. One is *Un Psychoanalyste Engagé*,[1] a book which initially was a series of conversations with a Swiss–Spanish colleague. The other one was François Dupare's *André Green*.[2] I don't mind doing it again.

GK   Good.

AG   I was born in Egypt in 1927, in Cairo. My father came from Alexandria, while my mother's family was established in Egypt from the fifteenth century; both came from a Sephardic background. My mother's maiden name was Barcilon. By the way, I have a cousin in New York whose name is José Barcilon. The history of my maternal family is well known; they had come from Spain and moved to Spanish Morocco, Tangier, and then they crossed all the borders, if there were any, along the shores of the sea, the Mediterranean and settled finally in Egypt, firstly in the delta of the Nile, and in the end in Cairo and Alexandria.

GK   This was a direct consequence of the Inquisition.

AG   Yes. In contrast, my father's family's history is much more obscure to us, for different reasons. My father never spoke much of his own family. Most of his family were in Alexandria. We lived in Cairo. He had a sister in Cairo but he did not have much contact with the part of the family that remained in Alexandria. His family had Spanish and Portuguese origins. My father understood Spanish but did not speak it, while my mother did. How they came about to be in Egypt is more mysterious. There is a family story saying that they had been in Hungary, so they probably came from the other side, through Europe, Western Europe, they went down via Turkey and the Middle East and arrived in Egypt. Well, this is the official story. I know that my father had cousins who were wealthier than he was, and it is thanks to them that my name now is spelt 'Green' because they added an 'e' to the original name which was 'Gren'. Nothing to do with 'Grinberg' or 'Greenman'. I have never encountered that name anywhere else. One of my father's cousins, who probably was a bit snobbish, decided to add an 'e' to make it sound more English and all the other Grens decided this was a good idea and did the same. Since *when* my father's family was in Egypt, it is difficult to know. Anyhow, life in Egypt was a very special thing. There was a very strong French influence in Egypt, which probably started with Bonaparte's expedition in 1799. If, for instance, you read French literature, all the great French writers had their trip to the Orient with a relatively lengthy stay in Egypt – Chateaubriand, Flaubert, Nerval, many others. And they all gave accounts of very pleasant memories from Egypt. There was the Arabic community and the European community, and although the English were important in politics and in administration, the common language of all the so-called Europeans in fact was not Arabic, but French. The culture was cosmopolitan but the language and the strongest influence came from France. The strongest impetus was given later under Mehmed Ali, who was francophile. I have memories ... I have memories that may surprise some people. When my mother listened to the radio, for example, listened to the news saying that Paris had fallen to the German army, she cried. France was important for all of us. There were also special circumstances in my family, which explains why France was especially important. My eldest sister (who was 14 years older than me) was 14 when she had a disease which is called in French, *mal de Pott*, tuberculosis of the vertebral column, which was impossible to treat in Egypt at the time. This institution which specialised in the treatment of these diseases (which at that time lasted four years) was in France. So my sister was put in this institution in the north of France and she stayed there for four years. My mother was – like any mother whose daughter was away because of an illness – very sad and rather depressed and my parents used to go for holidays to France as soon as school stopped. They would spend two months there to enable my mother to stay with my sister. So, that was also a reason for France being important for my family before my birth.

GK   How many siblings did you have?

AG   I had three siblings. I had two sisters and one elder brother but I happened to be the accident of the family. I was born nine years after my elder brother, who was the youngest of the three, and, as I said, there were fourteen years between my elder sister and myself. The diagnosis of my mother's pregnancy was made in Paris and that's also a reason why France could have been important to me, unconsciously.

GK   What about your grandparents? Did you grow up in the context of a close, strong family within a large extended family?

AG   I didn't know any of my grandparents; my brother and sisters didn't know them either. I didn't know what a grandfather or grandmother meant. My father had little contact with his own family. When he went to Alexandria, he did visit his sister, especially one of his sisters; I believe there were seven. But my father had no strong ties with his family. My mother, that was totally different. She spoke with great respect and awe of her father, whom I imagined as a kind of scholar feared by everyone in the family. They were a very united family; she was all the time at her brother's house and her sister's home and so on. But I wouldn't say that in my own family, family life was very important. I had a special position, being the youngest. I had cousins of my age, who lived in Alexandria, but I saw them only in the summer when I used to go to Alexandria because of the sea and the resorts by the sea. But even then ... I only had one cousin who I used to see frequently. Although we were Jewish, Sephardic Jews, it was a paradoxical situation: while Jewishness was absolutely affirmed, there was no religious practice whatsoever. I never knew what a Shabbat was. We were Jews at Yom Kippur; we went to the synagogue on Rosh Hashana, Yom Kippur, and Passover. There is a legend that when I was born, my father went to the synagogue and when he heard the rabbi singing *Eliyahu ha-Navi*, towards the end of the Sabbath service, he decided that my name would be Elijah, but unfortunately he did not register it. My father was not a religious person but two years before he died — and he knew he would die soon because he had a serious illness — a rabbi came home to teach him Hebrew, so he may have wanted to be ...

GK   ... at peace with the Almighty, after all.

AG   Yes, all clear before he died ... You know, friends were important, very important. When I arrived in Europe it was a considerable change for me, because in Egypt I was at home in any of my friends' homes. I could come at any time, leave at any time, share the meal, and be considered a member of the family. There was no question about this. When I arrived in France I think it took one year before anyone invited me to his or her home. People who wanted to see me saw me in the café.

GK   What age are we talking about then; when did you go to Paris, and why?

AG   Well, important things happened in my family. First, I lost my father when I was 14, not yet 14. Both of my parents died at 59, and there was a difference, eight years difference, between my father and my mother. They both died, so I was 14 when my father died; by then, the financial situation of the family wasn't good at all. My father had had a lot of money, but because of my sister's illness, he had to accompany my mother when she came to Europe. Also, her cure in France was very expensive; it lasted four years. That meant that his job was out of his control for two months every time. He lost his good financial position.

The last years of my father's life were not very happy in terms of his professional career, though he was a very intelligent man whose intelligence was recognised by others. After his death, my family didn't know what they were going to do. Part of my family wished me to go into business in order to work as soon as possible, to help the family. But I was good at school and one sister saw how sad I was (she had also suffered because her studies had been interrupted too soon) and she decided to take on my defence and to convince the family that I should continue till the *baccalauréat*, which I did. And then something else happened. I fell ill at the last year, not the last year, it was the year before the last one, and I couldn't go to school. I had to stay in bed all the time but I still prepared my examination, the first part of the *baccalauréat*, and I succeeded. My family was impressed and decided to help me. I got a scholarship for half and the family helped me with the other half. Finally, I went to France at the age of 19, the year that coincided with the end of the war and the start of university. But to tell you the truth, I had it in mind to go to Europe under any circumstance long before. I went there to do my studies, but I hadn't decided yet *what* to do. One rich uncle gave me an amount of money, saying to me that he had done something for each of my brother and sisters, he hadn't done anything for me, and so he decided to give me a certain sum and left me free to use it as I wanted. It was my responsibility and I decided to use that money for studying, but still I had to decide what to study. My inclination would have been to study philosophy but as I wasn't French, I had no nationality, there was no point. The only way to earn a living with philosophy is to teach, and if you have no nationality and if you haven't got the right diplomas, you can't do that. So I gave up that idea pretty quickly.

GK   No nationality? Presumably you had an Egyptian passport?

AG   No, no.

GK   How did you travel?

AG   *Apatride*! I was a stateless person. My father, after having been in Egypt for many generations, thought that we would be granted nationality automatically. He was wrong. Now, philosophy, you see, was out of the question. I decided maybe I can do some kind of scientific studies but I was discouraged from doing this. One of my uncles said, 'What are you going to do? Are you going to analyse *ka-ka* and *pee-pee* all your life? It's not interesting, don't do that, it's absurd.' And finally I made a bet; I took up a challenge, because you can't call that otherwise, it was a bet. I said, 'I'm going to do medicine', having already in mind that I would become a psychiatrist. I never wanted to be a general practitioner.

GK   Why psychiatry? How did you come to this decision?

AG   Here, of course, we start the analysis. I believe that the dead mother is a paper which has been valued not only because of its clinical findings, but because it is linked to a personal experience. When I was 2 years old, my

13

mother had a depression: she had a younger sister, who died after having been burned accidentally. She was the youngest sister of the family, my Aunt Rose, and my mother got depressed. I have seen photographs – one can tell from her face that she had really a very severe depression. At that time, treatment was very poor. She went to rest in a thermal station near Cairo. I can only suppose that I have been very strongly marked by this experience which, of course, needed three analyses to relive fully. This must have been the reason, because I remember a conversation I had with a friend of my father when I was 12, in which I said already then that I wanted to study the mental diseases.

GK   Your mother had gone away, who looked after you? Your sisters? Do you know?

AG   At that time the family situation was still good, financially. When I was young we had European nurses, mostly Italian.

GK   Italian? Not French?

AG   No, no, no. You know, the French in Egypt were a special colony; they usually did not live in Cairo. They lived in the canal area. They were people from the canal administration; they lived in Port Said. Those who lived in Cairo and Alexandria were either teachers (who taught in the French institutions) or were working with the embassy, the consulate, the cultural politics of France. So we had no French governess; the governesses were usually Italian or, in some very highbrow families, English nurses. So the person who looked after me must have been an Italian governess *and* my two sisters. When the family lost part of its wealth my sister took care of me. My sister stopped school at 14. I was 12 years younger. She was a second mother to me as I was 2 years old when she left school. My father had already financial problems because of my older sister's illness.

GK   So you go to Paris to study medicine, wanting to do psychiatry. What year do you arrive in Paris?

AG   1946.

GK   The war had just ended.

AG   I took the second boat that made the connection between Egypt and Marseilles; when we arrived in Marseilles we had to wait for four days until we could take the train to Paris. I arrived in Paris on the 8th of May and I remember there was a celebration of the victory.

GK   A very special time to arrive to Paris.

AG   Yes, it was a special time. Paris was not completely out of the war. Of course, there was peace; yes, 1946 – it was the first anniversary, but still there was nothing to eat, you had to have vouchers for everything. But this was not the main thing – parents always care for their poor children's food. This was not important to us. What was most important for us was how very isolated we all felt. It was such a difference coming from Egypt, where everybody knew everybody. We didn't possess a colonial mentality because we knew that we were not 'the masters of the land'. The masters were the British, as far as foreigners were concerned, or the *pashas*, the wealthy landowners; these were the masters. But, of course, we were the privileged Europeans who could benefit from the European educational system; we belonged to a kind of closed society, but we were not the masters.

GK   What kind of school did you attend? You mentioned the *baccalauréat*.

AG   There were all sorts of schools. There was an English school, for those who wanted to send their children to England or to have an English education. There was an Italian school, which was a very good school, and just as the communities had their own hospitals – the Greeks had their hospitals, the Italians had their hospitals, the Americans had theirs – they also had their schools. As far as the French were concerned, there were two types of school, and this was a capital difference between the two: one was religious, the Brothers of Saint Mark. The other was the French *laque* school; we felt in the *laque* school that we were really at the top of the world; we were not religious and we were *French*, we were the *l'esprit de la République française*.

GK   You arrive in Paris, feeling French but an *apatride*, a Jew with no passport wanting to go to university. Was it easy to get in the university then?

AG   It was automatic, just as it is today. The problem was that I had made myself ... illusioned. I thought that as soon as I arrived in France, I immediately would be in contact with the young French intellectuals. Nothing of the kind happened, of course. When I arrived on Boulevard Saint Michel and tried to see where 'the young French intellectuals' were, I couldn't see anybody. It was a feeling of complete isolation, a feeling of being lost in the crowd, the Paris crowd, a crowd of poor students. I had also a lot of ambivalence on my part about medicine. I wanted to become a psychiatrist from the beginning; I knew that I could not see a psychiatric patient before four to five years, so I had to wait, and I had to suffer. The teaching of medicine was *very* boring. For the first years, I was a bad student. I didn't pay much attention to my exams and I used to work for myself; I studied philosophy, psychology; I read books about culture, not very useful for my medical training.

GK   Hanna Arendt makes the distinction somewhere between Judaism and Jewishness; she argues that there has been an important, fundamental change in history: Jews have kept an identity as Jews; they might be in touch with their Jewishness, but they have lost their religiosity, their Judaism. When you arrived to Paris in 1946, was there any relevance in your being Jewish?

AG   Yes. I knew, of course, that there still was anti-Semitism in France, as it has always been. But one must say that during those times, anti-Semitism was not so evident as it had been before and during the war. The war was very recent and we knew about concentration camps; people were still shocked. When I think of myself back then, my Jewish identity was unimportant for me. I didn't specially look for Jews, or non-Jews. I was still in contact with the Jewish friends who had come from Egypt; we used to live in the same hotel, seeing each other, going into each other's rooms, and chatting and having meals together sometimes. When I started to go to the university, this was the first opportunity to meet a true mixture of people, some Jews and some non-Jews; I must say, personally, I always had good relationships with all of them. Now, one day, I met a young girl who I found very attractive and I invited her to go out to the theatre or something like that, and she said to me, 'I'm not allowed to go out with young men who have not been presented to my parents.' I said I didn't mind, that I was ready to meet her parents. And that's where she replied, 'It's impossible for me to bring you home because you are Jewish.' So that was the first time, and I must say, the unique time in which somebody told me that I was excluded from something because of being a Jew. I was somehow shocked, but I recovered from it. The great change, again, was when I won the *concours*. I don't know if you know about it, but there is a system in France of *concours* …

GK   It's like a competition for a post, say in a hospital …

AG   Sainte Anne's hospital was a special place in Paris. In all Paris hospitals, general hospitals, the tradition was more or less conservative; medical people were on the right of the political spectrum. Young doctors came from the bourgeoisie, but Sainte Anne had an entirely different background and tradition. Sainte Anne, the Mecca of psychiatry, was leftist, not communist, but for the left. We were the intellectuals. You know, there was a tradition in these *salles de garde*. The paintings on the walls of these *salles de garde* were all pornographic; the more pornographic, the more typically medical. Sainte Anne's *salle de garde* was different. The walls were covered by paintings that had been made by surrealist painters; the theme was not the illustration of some pornographic songs that they used to sing, for example, like in other places. The theme of these paintings was trying to match themes from psychiatry and themes dear to surrealism. And they were of very great quality. Painters like Oscar Dominguez, Jacques Hérold, Maurice Henry, and others who were well-known surrealist painters, had painted these walls. Unfortunately, they had to be later destroyed because we had to move to another building; we lived for four years in that setting; it was very stimulating for us, we were so proud of it. The fact that politically we were on the left was only one aspect of the picture; we were also standing, intellectually, on the revolutionary side, surrealism and so on. Anti-Semitism could not be a problem in Sainte Anne. Henri Ey's wife was Jewish; Lacan's wife was Jewish too, and many, many others. I cannot say that I have even heard any kind of remark about being Jewish or not; the problem of Jewish identity was never a problem to me. My first wife was a non-Jew. She was Orthodox on her father's side, Catholic on her mother's side; my children had no religious education at all. So what remains of my Jewishness? I can tell you that in 1948, when the first war started between Egypt and Israel, there I reacted to it. I felt for Israel, I worried about it, I was very concerned about this country being surrounded by all these Arab enemies ... this is really the problem with Jewish people who are not religious: they forget they are Jewish till the day the Jews are threatened, persecuted, or anything of the kind anywhere, and yet, on the other hand, we do not agree at all with the politics of Israel.

GK   What about later on, when you got into contact with Lacan? I was surprised to hear some Lacanian analysts – not in France, I must add – talked at times in ways that suggested hints of anti-Semitism ...

AG   Lacan, no, no, no, I would even say the contrary. Lacan suffered from ... not being Jewish! Of course, I am joking. The situation with him was complicated, but what I said has a grain of truth. I have written – and I am not the only one to have made the observation – that Lacan's psychoanalysis is a Christian version of it. But I cannot say that I ever heard anything in Lacan about that. There had been rumours that while he was in conflict with his colleagues from the International he may have said something, but I personally never heard Lacan say anything. My life totally changed because maybe I wasn't part of the French intellectual class, but being at Sainte Anne's Hospital was a privilege; it was a very active centre of discussion, debate, encounters and meetings – a very dynamic institution.

GK   Who were the psychiatrists then? Who were the main figures?

AG   It's too bad we're not in Paris, I would have shown you lots of photographs. In 1953, I won that *concours*. The first year I went to a psychiatric hospital which was 40 kilometres out of Paris, where the conditions were very poor. I only stayed there for one year, and then immediately I came back to Sainte Anne's hospital, which is the equivalent of the Maudsley. Sainte Anne's Hospital was, for a young psychiatrist who wished to learn, an extraordinary place. Henry Ey was indisputably the most important figure of psychiatry in France, and maybe even in the world. His department was not in Sainte Anne; it was out of Paris, about 130 kilometres from Paris, near Chartres. I don't know whether you've heard of him ...

GK   I have. I studied psychiatry from his book, *Manuel de Psychiatrie*, which he wrote with Paul Bernard and Charles Brisset. That was *the* textbook in my psychology course, which I believe was quite unique then in Argentina, in the sense that we learned the French system of psychiatric classification.

AG   Well, I can say I was Henri Ey's favourite pupil, and when he retired
he asked me to continue his lectures. And I even did it for some time,
and then I gave up. I gave it up because I said, 'Look, let's be honest, I'm
not a psychiatrist.' Every day I became more of a psychyoanalyst; I could
not pretend I could teach psychiatry; being as I am, this was not me. I
can't pretend to be something that I'm not. Ey had started his own career
by being a resident in Sainte Anne's in the 1920s. He ended his psychiatric training in 1926. He was a close friend of Lacan's and also to one of
my other masters, who is not really known beyond the frontiers of
France, Pierre Male, who was a most important child psychiatrist. After
the split in 1953, Male and Lacan, belonging to different societies, never
met again. Male was on the side of Nacht, but Lacan and Ey remained
friends to the end. The Paris Society had been created in 1927. After a
while, as you know, Rudy Lowenstein came to Paris, and Hartmann too.
Rudy Lowenstein settled in France and analysed four important people:
Nacht, Lacan, Lagache, and Pierre Male. Ey wanted to build and develop
a new psychiatry. He wanted to include psychoanalysis in a broader
view, which also included phenomenology, the biological findings, and
so on. Lacan, while being a close friend, was also a rival. Ey's influence
was purely moral because he wasn't a professor of psychiatry. He used to
come every week to teach and then he would go back to his *abbaye*.
People went to Ey only to learn something from him; they didn't expect
to get anything else from him. With Lacan, it was different; he wanted
people to come to him like a spider; he would analyse them, make them
his pupils, attach them to his person, and finally turn them into apostles.

GK   Henri Ey never really wanted to become a psychoanalyst, but he was to
psychiatry in France what Lacan in the end was for psychoanalysis. Nevertheless, psychoanalysis remained for Ey a footnote, a bit like in his
Manuel, in the text ...

AG   It was much more polemic than a footnote. His position was, 'yes, yes,
of course there is something called the unconscious but there is something much more important which was consciousness'. In his view of
consciousness, consciousness is containing and repressing and controlling
the unconscious, whenever the unconscious took hold of consciousness
then disease developed. He wanted to ensure the primacy of consciousness in what he called – and psychiatry was called by him (and this you
will understand) – 'pathology of freedom'. Being sane was having the
possibility of being free. If the unconscious took hold of the person, then
we have the pathology of freedom; the individual was caught in this
conflict, and so on. To this, he added the biological causes. This is how
he developed his strange theory, his 'organo-dynamism' – organo, because of the biological background; dynamism, because it belonged to
the dynamics of psychic life. He was the Pope of psychiatry. We have
this tradition in France that once a year we have what we call a *dîner de*

patron – dinner for the bosses – at which all the chiefs of wards and departments are invited, and the residents laugh at them, they imitate them; everybody enjoys that – this is once a year. I was Pope Henry once. It was true that he was the Pope of psychiatry because he was a person of an enormous vitality and scholarship; he used to organise meetings on important problems. For instance, one in 1947 was on *the psychogenesis of psychosis and neurosis* – Lacan gave an important paper there.

GK   That was the Bonneval *colloquium*, wasn't it? Lacan presented 'Propos sur la causalité psychique' ...

AG   That's right. It's a place near Chartres, 130 kilometres, and at which we stayed for a week. It was an abbey which was turned into a hospital.

GK   In the last Bonneval *colloquium*, on *The Unconscious*, that was the first time I came across your name. You presented 'The unconscious and psychopathology', and wrote an introductory chapter, called 'The doors of the unconscious', for the publication of the papers.

AG   That's right.

GK   At any rate, Ey was a very important figure, a rather benign one ...

AG   He was a man who was childless; we were all his children. And, apart from my own real father, he was truly the only father figure that I ever had. Lacan was not a father figure. He was a man I admired; I was fascinated by him. But I could never think of him as a father figure. At a distance, Bion was a father figure, but not Lacan. We had a lot of affection for Henry because he treated us with great respect. Even the most insignificant resident could raise his hand and say, 'I don't agree with you because of this, this and this'. And Henry would listen and he would answer. He had, of course, temper tantrums like many people in that position. But he adored human exchanges ... Of course, some people would say he would pervert the game between the Lacanians and the non-Lacanians. But that's not true. He loved discussion, and he loved to create debates. If there was an opportunity for debates between Lacanians and non-Lacanians he would use it. Debating was the important thing.

GK   Intellectual debate, the influence of the intellectual *milieu*, philosophy, the humanities, all of that seems to have been always important in France.

AG   But you can't say it didn't happen in other countries because you have the example of Germany. One could argue that the history of European psychiatry – and I don't want to offend my British colleagues – is a struggle of giants between the French and the Germans. They accuse each other of being obscure and lacking rigour and so on, but there was the idea since the beginning, since the classical authors of the nineteenth century, that there are philosophical grounds and consequences drawn from the consideration of mental disease. Pinel, the great liberator, wrote a *Traité médico-philosophique de l'aliénation mentale*, the idea that philosophy is in the background was very deeply rooted. Since psychiatry has become 'active', this has changed. Before this time, psychiatrists had little to do, so there were two types of psychiatrists: those who did nothing and really did nothing, and those who were very active in thinking, writing, observing. This is an entire period of naturalistic observation of what mental diseases are, *and* philosophical conclusions which were drawn from the study of the brain. From this you have the earliest statistics, and the classification of mental diseases. It took centuries to arrive at a classification which could stand on its feet and be consistent; all sorts of classifications preceded the ones that we use now. In my first years of training I read a lot of these books. It's difficult to imagine the richness of the observations that are included in the old books. There were all sorts of treatments of course; one could see that there were the sadistic ones, and others that were more humanistic. But the history of psychiatry is still something very, very interesting, and when we had Ey as a teacher he always included a view on the history of psychiatry and the philosophical questions. There was reciprocity between the different disciplines. Sartre's influence I remember quite well; his book *Critique de la Raison Dialectique* was published just before the Bonneval *colloquium* on the unconscious. He was now in his prime. Merleau-Ponty was important and much more crucial to psychoanalysis. Merleau-Ponty's wife, Suzanne, had been in analysis with Lacan and became a psychoanalyst of the Lacanian school. Merleau-Ponty used to teach in the Sorbonne. He very much wanted to come to Paris to teach. He was first in Strasbourg, I believe. I don't remember in what province he used to teach, but the only Chair available for him was the Chair of Child Psychology. So he taught child psychology, even though he knew nothing about it. But he gave a very interesting seminar, comparing Anna Freud and Melanie Klein, which was the first time this happened in the Sorbonne. Lagache was already there. Merleau-Ponty gave a course on Saussure in 1951; even before Lacan, he directed our attention to Saussure. Then, there was Lévi-Strauss, and Paul Ricoeur.

GK   You mention Lagache in passing. Lagache was also a very important, influential person. And yet, he was always a strange figure in French psychoanalysis for me.

AG   Yes, because it is difficult to place him. Lagache was, first, *élève de l'Ecole Normale supérieure*. He was professor of psychology in the Sorbonne. Being a psychiatrist, he had no real inclination for psychiatry. He was in the tradition of people who, when they want to teach psychopathology in the Sorbonne, had to have some kind of training in psychiatry. He did that quite well and then he also became a psychoanalyst. His main function was as a teacher: he taught psychology, psychopathology, social psychology. There was a very strong rivalry between him and Nacht and he was at the centre of the first split. Until 1953 there was no training institute; there was the Society, which had a training committee just as you have. But in 1953 *L'Institut de psychanalyse* was created; it was in charge of all the problems of training, being an independent institution from the Society. Lagache, as professor in the Sorbonne, thought that he was the one who should run this thing. Nacht wouldn't let him; Nacht had the idea and the hope of becoming a professor of psychoanalysis in the faculty of medicine – a hope which any reasonable person wouldn't have had, knowing the state of mind of the professors. And there were many people who supported him in the Institute. He had his clique: Lebovici, and many others. So the two came into conflict. The conflict, of course, was about an unimportant matter, and finally Lagache decided to quit. And wherever Lagache would go, others would go too because some depended on him for their career at the university. Lacan and Lagache formed the French Society in which they co-existed for ten years, from 1953 to 1963. When the problem with the IPA took place, because of Lacan's short sessions, Rudy Lowenstein – who thought very well of Lagache – recommended him highly; Hartmann had a great appreciation of his work and if you read Lagache there is a Hartmannian flavour in it. These people had to solve an impossible problem: how to accept Lagache, while leaving Lacan out. It took them at least five or six years to solve the problem which ended in the second split. In the French Society, after the split with the Paris Society, there weren't so many training analysts and people who could supervise, so most of them had their analysis with Lacan and their supervisions with Lagache.

GK   When did you come to analysis?

AG   After 1953. When I won my *concours*, I resisted psychoanalysis for another three years. I was very biologically oriented, psychiatrically oriented; my masters at the time were Ey and also a man – I don't know how much you've heard of him – Ajuriaguerra. He was a neurologist and a psychiatrist and he studied child development and I was also one of his favourite pupils. It was finally him who told me, 'You should really go to analysis', because I really had a very bad temper, which by the way I have managed to keep – with slight improvement, I hope. I started my analysis in 1956, for four years, with Maurice Bouvet, who was considered one of the best in the Paris Society. There was the authority of Nacht, and after him there was Bouvet. Bouvet hesitated, but finally he decided to stay with Nacht. I had my analysis from 1956 to 1960 and the last time I saw my analyst was my very last session, because he died afterwards.

GK   The last session! Had you known he was ill?

AG   Other people knew he was ill. I was the only one not to know. I thought it was all projections ...

GK   So, you started your analysis, but that doesn't make you necessarily interested in analysis.

AG   True. In the first three years I kept on studying psychiatry very hard and that's how I got a kind of cultural background, not only in psychiatry but also in neurology, which I took with Ajuriaguerra. Sainte Anne's offered so many opportunities! Psychoanalysts were very influential then, and I was able to attend their consultations, among them, Lacan. I could see how they proceeded, I was attracted by that, realising very quickly that each one had his own originality, his own specificity, his own approach, and that one could not talk of 'one' psychoanalysis. And of course, when they gave courses, I attended them. I became progressively involved, and Lacan started an enormous game of seduction towards me. One of my best friends was Rosolato, who was in analysis with him. And Lacan would take any opportunity to get in touch with me *through* him. One day Lacan even gave him a reprint of his to pass on to me. In 1958 there was a Congress of Psychotherapy in Barcelona which Ey and Lacan attended. I met Lacan there, and he invited me to have a drink at his hotel. I went with Rosolato; for two hours Lacan tried to exert pressure on me: 'Why don't you come with me, you should be at my right.' I said to him, 'Look, what you write is of great interest to me, but I need people to teach me my profession, and in balance, if I put you on one side and I put all the others who can teach me on the other side ... it goes this way.' He was furious that he could not be heavier than at least the sum of six rivals. And Rosolato was there; he was in analysis with Lacan. You know, Lacan was totally cynical. People do not know him; he was totally cynical. He wouldn't care at all that Rosolato was there. That was his way. He forced Rosolato into that position of jealousy, resentment, and everything that you can imagine in such a situation. Would I had been in Rosolato's position, I think I could not have avoided feeling as I suppose he must have felt.

GK   From outside, at a distance, there was something not only seductive but also psychopathic ...

AG   Sure. A person who hasn't known Lacan and seen him in action cannot imagine what it was like with him. He was fascinating. He had an extraordinary intelligence, and he could also be very kind. He had a perverse character, which was absolutely obvious, but people wouldn't see it. The general opinion was, 'You cannot judge Lacan with the same tools with which you judge other people because he is a *genius*'.

GK   Where is Rosolato now?

AG   He is an important member of the French Society, very influential, one of the four most important people.

GK   I found his writings very inspiring. One paper, which I remember with particular interest, is the one on 'The Narcissistic Axis of Depression'.

AG   Yes, it's one of his good papers. This was a period that was very important to us, which started in 1970, 1972, the period of the *Nouvelle Revue de psychanalyse*. At that time, Pontalis decided to create the *Revue* with the collaboration of the people from the French Association (which took over after the disappearance of the French Society where Lacan and Lagache co-existed), but keeping its own independence. I joined the Editorial Board in 1972. For all of us, it became a landmark in the history of French psychoanalysis, because it is really what helped us to liberate ourselves from Lacan: we discovered the British analysts, and Masud Khan was asked to be the British editor. When I think of my own work, I realised recently that I have been wrong. I thought that I had a Lacanian period, and afterwards a British period. And when I looked at the dates, I saw that I had been mistaken. 1961 was the year in which I started to attend Lacan's seminars, but it was in fact the same year that I attended the first pre-congress in London, before the Edinburgh congress, and I met then most of the British colleagues I happen to know today. I attended seminars by Winnicott, John Klauber and Herbert Rosenfeld; I had made my choice, and it was a good choice! I was very, very impressed; for the first time I had the feeling that, here there were people who taught me something close to my experience; it opened my eyes, it was something I hadn't heard before. The influence of the British on my thinking was, in fact, parallel to the one of Lacan, with the difference that I had Lacan every week, while I had the British every six months.

GK   When did you write the book on affects? What year was that?

AG   1970. It was not planned to be a book. You know, we have something which is very specific to the Paris Society, we have the Congress of Romance Languages. For this event, reporters are designated. *Reporters* are not at all what you mean by reporters, when you usually use that word in English. Reporters write a report, but a report was frequently 150 pages long, which will be used in the future as reference, a sort of monograph. If you want to know something about a problem, a question, to find out about the bibliography on a particular subject, then you go to this report, and even if you don't agree with what is said you can find the information which is useful to you, which you will use for your work. So I wrote, in fact, more than a report; I wrote, I think it was 300 pages, and it was initially called *L'Affect*. As you know, I had stopped all relations with Lacan when I quarrelled with him in 1967. I had been with him for seven years and I then stopped. I decided to write something because the argument on affect was already present in my discussion of Laplanche's and Leclaire's paper on the unconscious, in Bonneval in 1960. When Lacan read it, he was totally furious. He called it 'the abject'. He understood that the criticism was centred on his work, and three years after the report I transformed it into a book – only the title had changed. It was published under the more appealing title, *Le Discours vivant*.

GK   As far as I remember, at the time in Argentina, where I was still living (I moved to London in 1970), it came as a surprise to many to hear of your separation from Lacan. We didn't have much information about what was really going on in Paris …

AG   But, to speak of Argentina, Baranger was French and he had maintained a relationship with the French analysts. He used to go every year to France and attended Lacan's seminar. He invited to come to Buenos Aires, first, Leclaire, and the year after he invited me. I stayed there two weeks. Baranger was perfectly aware that by that time I was separated from Lacan, I was no longer with the Lacanians. But this was later; my visit was in 1974.

GK   Where did you write about the Christianity of his ideas?

AG   It's a paper, quite a lengthy paper (in fact, it has the format of a book), which has been included in a book, *Language in Psychoanalysis* – a criticism of Lacan's ideas. Lacan cheated everybody in saying, 'Let's return to Freud'. It wasn't a bad idea, obviously, the psychoanalytical ideas that were active at that time came from the Americans: the ego, and adaptation; something had to be done. Lacan fought against this, and I think that he was right, and other people and I continue fighting against these views – even at the risk of my relationship deteriorating with my American colleagues. In any case, the return to Freud was interesting because there was the feeling that he had been misunderstood. But the return to Freud was an excuse, it just meant going to Lacan. This return to Freud was in fact a trick. You know, it is difficult to say if it was deliberate, or it was something that he wanted to promote and finally realised himself that the whole thing turned against him. Of course, there are different Freuds. There is the purely psychological Freud, the Freud of the unconscious, the Freud of the metapsychology, the Freud of the beautiful papers like the one on fetishism, and so on. This is the purely psychological Freud. But there is also the consideration (which becomes stronger and stronger in Freud's view) of the biological roots of the mind. This, Lacan wouldn't buy at all. If you study the Freudian theoretical system, you see that it is impossible to leave one aside, and try to keep the other; you have to rebuild it entirely; that's what the little book by Gilbert Diatkine[3] is so good about: he shows exactly and precisely how, in fact, Lacan is in contradiction with Freud on many, many issues. The question of language, for instance: Lacan saying that the unconscious is structured like a language. As I have already shown, when you read Freud, it is obvious that this proposition doesn't work for a minute. Freud very clearly opposes the unconscious (which he says is constituted by thing-representations and nothing else) to the pre-conscious. What is related to language can only belong to the pre-conscious; Lacan tried to defend himself by emphasising that he said 'like a language', but that's not true. In other instances, he says the unconscious *is* language. He even says, in some places, that the real person who invented the theory of the unconscious is not Freud but Lacan, as if Freud had a vague intuition of it, but really the rigorous definition came from him. Then, if you come to the idea of the Name of the Father, the Name of the Father is a Christian concept, because what he wants to say is that it is not the father which is important, it is the instance of the father, the dead father, the ancestor, which is an interesting idea. But as he wants to bring the law into the system, instead of the superego, then he has to invoke the Name of the Father: in the Name of the Father, the Son, and the Holy Spirit, and so on. We must not forget his relationship with his brother, who was a Benedictine monk; Lacan had always had an ambiguous attitude towards religion. He would criticise the institutions of Christianity, but he would refer to *les pères de l'église*. Paul Roazen had an interview with the brother of Lacan shortly before he died. It was very interesting. One thing is sure: the relationship between the two brothers was very close. You may not know that Lacan tried to see the Pope, to have an interview with him. He didn't succeed. We know from Lacan's biography that Lacan was very, very sad when his brother told him that he decided to become a monk. And I know, because Lacan told me, how much he praised the work of his brother, Mark, to whom his thesis is dedicated. Of course, this biographical information is not enough, and must be completed by a detailed examination of his work. I have pointed out the influence of Augustine and Pascal in his work.

GK   Whatever we might think about some of Lacan's ideas, it is clear that he was brilliant: after having read Lacan, reading Freud has never been the same experience. Not necessarily because of the interpretations Lacan made of Freud's text, but the fact that he actually forced the reader to *interpret* Freud. That has been an amazing achievement: the importance of his proposal to return to Freud, was the re-interpreting of Freud.

AG   Yes. It is important, and I think all this is linked to the question of language. From the minute Lacan decided that what was important in psychoanalysis was language, he killed two birds with one stone. On the one hand, he developed a very strong argument: in the analytic cure, we proceed using only words and language. If we achieve something through this, then the structure of language and the structure of the unconscious must have something in common. This argument is very strong, but I can also demonstrate that it is wrong, that it is only the intersections of the two worlds, the unconscious and the pre-conscious, which makes language work. This is a way to reach, indirectly, the unconscious – even if the unconscious has nothing to do with the structure of language. Lacan was not only in agreement with the structuralist movement (which was based on the principle that the relationship between the elements is more important than the elements themselves) but also he brought something important from the Christian religion, that is,

the *verb*. 'In the beginning was the verb [*Editor's note*: it is *word* in Eng-
lish] and the verb was made flesh' – this is St John's Gospel, I'm translat-
ing from the French! One day, in a seminar, Lacan said this is the wrong
translation: one shouldn't say, 'In the beginning was the verb' but 'In the
beginning was speech' – *la parole*. A theologian who was in the audience
objected and said to him, 'I'm sorry, this is impossible, this cannot hold.'
Lacan was infuriated. Even for someone who is not trained in theology
like myself, it is clear that to use the verb is something quite different.
The verb is that part of language that refers to action; using the verb to
qualify the action still has close links with what it says; the verb becoming flesh is incarnation. It's a very strong and powerful image, but you
cannot do that with other parts of language. You cannot do that with
nouns or pronouns or adverbs, and so on. So it is not the question of
speech, it is really that part of speech which is related to action, that
which represents action, and probably more precisely with will. Lacan's
understanding of language is full of ambiguities. On one hand, it is a
formalistic approach, like the structuralist one was. On the other hand –
though claiming to be materialistic and claiming to be scientific – it is
mystical.

GK   You mentioned the question of the cure, and its relation to language,
in other words, the question of what is it that we are doing when practising psychoanalysis? What does a cure consist of? If we take the British
schools – even though it's so difficult to speak in terms of 'the British' ...

AG   But there is a British spirit ...

GK   Indeed. Now, in very general terms, one could argue that while the
British have given predominance to the *presence* of the analyst in the
process of the cure (and that has produced enormous progress in psychoanalytic technique), the French have focused their attention on the *absence* of the analyst ...

AG   There are reasons for that. Your distinction is quite accurate. For the
British, there is no question: psychoanalysis is a treatment. People come
to us for some reason, obviously not always for the same reason, but one
could argue, for example, because they have had a distorted development, and what you have to do is to cure them. I hope my British colleagues will still accept to talk to me after this characterisation. The
analyst is there to repair something. They are there to heal something in
the patient, to treat them, for example, like a nurse attending a dying
baby. They have to be ready to face, and sometimes to provoke, what is
most dangerous for the health of the child in order to fight ... what?
Here you have an important choice: the disease ... or evil! The notion of
evil may shock many of my British colleagues, but I cannot help thinking
that many analysts who belong to the British Society are very much
influenced by religious minds. They may not be officially religious but, as
I said one day, the difference between the British and the French, is that

the Catholics are supposed to stay bachelors, they are not supposed to have children; they may have children, but then they are illegitimate. British clergymen can have children, and they raise children in that spirit. This seems to be a joke, but it's serious. Think of all the analysts from your Society who have had a great influence of religion in their background. I think that the British analysts have great qualities; above all, they take responsibility for their patients. I do not think, for instance, that Lacanian practice could be very successful in England. People would be too shocked, too guilty; they would feel too dishonest to practise Lacanian analysis. But, on the other hand (and maybe this is an excuse I try to find for myself) I believe that five times a week sometimes leads to a kind of moral treatment and to a process of suggestion. Think also of the systematic interpretations of the weekend separations. There is a shared assumption that the patient needs the constant presence of a nurse to deal with a possible disaster any minute. This is in contradiction to the concept of the unconscious as working through in the absence of the object (as in the paradigm of the dream). When Freud started with a daily session, this was not because the patient could not be left by himself but because analysis was considered a sort of mental hygiene.

GK   I disagree with you on this one. I'm still a great believer in full analysis, but then, I have always been a supporter of it. When I was involved with the anti-psychiatry movement, in the early 1970s, I was even then practising five times a week analysis with schizophrenics and psychotic patients – although the culture around me didn't think much of it. Of course, it's not the only thing I practise …

AG   I believe that it is very linked to what you referred to before, the question and the dialectics of absence and presence. To my mind, a patient needs to breathe in between two sessions; he has to be able to re-organise his self and his defences.

GK   That's fine, but why would you think that they cannot do that from one day to the next, that they need 'an extra day' to achieve it? Of course, I think there is a distortion, and maybe an abuse in the discussion about five times a week: not all patients need, or for that matter can stand, full analysis. There is the mistaken belief that the more disturbed the patient, the more sessions he needs. In my experience, I have sometimes found that disturbed patients can only have a few sessions a week, even once a week. I also object to some of my colleagues when they seem to suggest that the only thing that counts is five times a week analysis. But let's go back to your argument for now.

AG   The second thing I would like to emphasise is the general ground of theory. The general ground of theory for me, as far as I can see, is a consequence of the too great importance that is given to child development. Everything is explained in terms of what has happened in the early phases. Melanie Klein goes back to six months; the non-Kleinians seem a little more flexible. I have just finished a paper today, for a symposium of the International (July 1998), where we're going to discuss 'temporality'. I have picked up ten items on temporality; all this has been reduced to – whatever you call it – developmental, maturational, genetic, whatever point of view. Entire blocks of utmost importance in Freud's theory are completely left out. It is not only the British; it's also the Americans. With the Americans it is sometimes the reverse of the British, focusing mainly on the ego, but it comes down to the same thing. They want to 'know' what has happened at six months and three days, and what happened at three years and two months and what happened at seven. They want a 'scale of development' that one could refer back to, they want to be able to follow the scale whenever one wants to ask a question. But, I say, what about timelessness in the unconscious? What about *Nachträglichkeit*? What do you do with primal fantasies? What do you think of the difference between timelessness in the unconscious and repetition-compulsion? Is it the same? Why isn't it the same? What do we think about drive theory? What is your approach? Your approach is psychological; do you think that your psychological approach accounts for some of the features that we find in repetition-compulsion, for instance? At Freud's death, the Ego psychologists pretended that they were Freud's heirs, but they couldn't cope with, or were unable to understand Freud's conception of time in psychoanalysis; it was too complicated for them. They left it out. And then they decided to observe! They would have the full scale of development; they would have liked to write the whole story, the life history of an individual, a total illusion! People do not function like that; most of the French don't see it like that. We have other points of disagreement that we need to debate. There is the naïve assumption that if you have registered all the *observable* events of a given period of time, then you will know what are the modifications, the changes taking place. It is exactly the contrary: *processes related to time are those that escape observation and most of them have to be deduced retrospectively.* Why? Because they took place intrapsychically, reorganising the results of perception, affects, phantasies, wishes, etc. This is the basis for transference to occur. Americans talk all the time of reconstructions. At the end of his life, Freud arrives at the conclusion that he has to give up the recovery of infantile amnesia, that some traumas have happened before the age of two or two-and-a-half, which cannot be recovered by memory: it can only be acted out or given an hallucinatory expression. So we have to lean on *construction*. Reconstruction means that you're going to find what was the real set of events which lead to the neurosis, but neurosis doesn't work like that, it isn't created this way. It develops in many different ways, going forward, backward, mixing up people and events. People haven't read Freud's paper on screen memories. It's all there, the idea of a linear concept of time is the most misleading idea; it is not by chance that a lot has been written about space, and nothing about time.

GK   As you know, I have myself argued against this linear concept of time. Anyhow, you mentioned space ...

AG   Space is very important, and the reason is very simple: it is because of the consulting room. The consulting room is a closed space. It is different from the outside space, and it is different, from what we can imagine, from inner space. It has a specificity of its own, and here is the point where Winnicott was a genius: he understood that in that space there is a transitional space which is touched by time; in the communication between the patient and the analyst the transitional space creates the possibility of a journey, the journey from inside to outside, a move to reach the real object coming from the object within. The object is created at the very moment that the subject is going to reach it in reality, just before he reaches it; it is created, and this is the subjective object. So the notion of a journey is important. Psychoanalytic theory has only one source, or at least an inescapable main source – the experience of what happens in the consulting room between the patient and the analyst. Let's take Bion, for instance. Bion described the capacity for reverie. Where did he learn about reverie? Obviously, not from observation. He learned it in the analytic situation: listening to the patient, trying to understand what the patient says, finally finding some sense while standing out of this communication, giving the interpretation to the patient, who seems to be stubborn, deaf, and it is then that he comes to the capacity for reverie of the mother, how it may happen or not happen. It was not because he had observed babies. How did Winnicott understand what was a transitional object? Because he was analysed, not because he observed babies; if he hadn't been analysed, he wouldn't have got a clue, and the idea wouldn't have occurred to him. You know, many of the infant researchers are not analysed – even if they had spent time on couches. It is really the analytic situation which is the frame and the model of *any* theory, *if* this theory is going to be considered a *psychoanalytic* theory. Applied psychoanalysis, OK, that's a different story. But psychoanalytic theory cannot be born out of observation, ever.

GK   No. I agree. Let's move on a bit. It seems to me that, together with the great preoccupation with – and the challenge offered by – the borderline cases that have invaded our clinical practices, psychoanalysts seem to have forgotten not only the neuroses but also something about madness. Madness was once at the centre of psychoanalytic thinking, your own collection in English was called *On Private Madness*. But that seems to have changed in the international literature. Winnicott, Bion, and many other great psychoanalytic writers understood madness well. At the core of Winnicott's thinking, giving a specific context to his theories, there is always the presence of a conflict: the conflict between the *fear of madness* and *the need to be mad*. To be alive is somehow to ride on the crest of this conflictual wave. This is also a kind of transitional space that one has to live in, between the fear and the need. Now, he was able to understand all this, what he did not seem to have taken into account were the drives, as if something was missing in his theory.

AG   I was very interested in this point. Madeleine Davis[4] wrote a book, where she tried to explain that Winnicott could not be considered as a full object relationship theoretician: to some extent, he believed also in drive theory. Drives were not, as Freud had said, what was in the beginning. In the beginning, Winnicott thought that the problems of coping with reality and helping the psyche to build its nest in the body were more important. And he gave an account, a very beautiful account of how the important thing for a baby is to find the possibility of experiencing his selfhood through omnipotence, the first exercise of subjectivity. He spoke of the *holding environment*, and of the possibility of creating the subjective object. This is what has to be ensured in every case in order to ensure a basic ground for the person, but then he added, 'if you want to have a really interesting personality, you have to link up with the drives'. You see how intelligent he was. The drives for him were indispensable: to have a creative personality, to have originality, to have something which gave you taste and flavour, you need the drives. I think you are right about fear of madness and the need to be mad. We have to link this with the change which has occurred between Freud and Winnicott. Freud showed the importance of illusion, but, in his mind, one had to fight illusion and accept disillusionment. Analysis was supposed to free the individual from his illusions, in favour of the dictatorship of reason and rationality. Winnicott says, 'You are wrong. Illusion is absolutely necessary for healthy development, you can only accept being disillusioned, if you have been *illusioned*'. Those who have not had the chance of being illusioned can only fail. Here of course we think of Winnicott's paper on the gaze of the mother, in which he speaks of the infants who cannot build a subjective object because they are all the time trying to look at the mother's face and to see what her reactions are, what are her feelings, if she approves, if she disapproves, and this, I think, is surely right. I agree totally. Up till now, I do not understand why, when I read Winnicott, I feel in total agreement with him, total. I believe that the problem about being mad or not being mad is probably linked to this thing, which is the journey. You know, the Greeks were great travellers, but there was one thing they feared the most: to lose the possibility of returning. So you can go very, very far away, but, if you're going to go mad, are you going to be able to return? I think Winnicott gave a much more convincing idea of what destruction is; he understood that destruction was not always destroying the object, destruction could also be the denial of the existence of the object. How many times do we have patients who would say, 'Who do you think you are? You do not exist.' In the end (especially where you get to the transference interpretations) some of them will then say, '*I* do not exist', which is something very close to their truth. And Winnicott recognises their right to aspire to that in the clinical situation.

GK We have been talking about the present pessimism about psychoanalysis. This seems to be happening at three different levels. There is the practical level, the lack of patients, the general crisis in psychoanalytic practice, which seems to originate in the difficulties in 'proving' the efficacy of psychoanalysis, the vulnerability that some psychoanalysts seemed to have felt with the critical attacks. There is also the theoretical pessimism: the contradictions inherent in our theories, the misunderstandings about what the theory is all about, is it about sexuality? Is it about objects? What is our understanding of the position of the analyst? There are many, many theoretical issues that need to be resolved, and this goes together with the feeling, and sometimes the conviction, that the theoretical differences cannot be resolved. And then there is also the problem of the institutions, which is another source of discontent, and of pessimism. At some level, this takes us back to Freud's own disappointment, and his statement about how little the psychoanalytic community has been changed by psychoanalysis.

AG I agree with you that the present situation is the result of a cumulative process, it appears as if all the denials which have been accumulated in the last decades have resurfaced, but the problems are very old. On the other hand, the dissatisfaction about lack of patients seems to be quite recent. How should we fight this? I'm afraid I have an opinion which many people will find too conservative, not on institutions but for instance on theory. Being 'too conservative' means that I am one of the last believers in Freud's theory. Not that I think we should take it as it is and repeat it as a bible. This has never been in my mind, I cannot be called an orthodox Freudian if I admire Winnicott, Bion and Lacan. If I admire these people, I necessarily admit that Freud is not enough. But let us say that I am very selective about the work of people which I really think should be studied and deepened. And let us say in passing how much I am surprised now that if one participates in any meeting and says three words, immediately people rush to have this published. What for? In three years' time nobody will ever read what an analyst said at that time, there is such an inflation of analytic literature, but it only shows a narcissistic infatuation – people think that what they have said has to be kept and memorised for future generations. This is totally silly; it cannot do much for psychoanalysis. People should be much more careful in publishing only what is worthwhile, what needs to be thought about, and reconsidered. So, what do I mean when I say that I consider that Freud's work is much more varied than people used to think? If you think of

Freud's theory, not only as a set of propositions which are articulated and which try to answer some questions which are not all clinical, some of them are related to the functioning of the mind as it appears in culture, in literature, in all the branches of knowledge where we suspect the unconscious to be, so if we take this, we see that what Freud was trying to match was some of his revolutionary ideas with the need for a general theoretical consistency.

Let us take an example: Freud's biological references. Today it is very fashionable to say that this is garbage. To remain on a theoretical ground: people say that these hypotheses are not valid at all, nobody has ever proved the existence of a drive, nobody has seen a drive, this – they say – is nineteenth-century speculation. All right. But if you say that, you have to face two questions. One, how is the mind connected to the body? Second, if you take it away, what are you going to replace it with? In England, in spite of the controversies, the opposition to Freud was not, I would say, mainly on a critical theoretical basis. One lady came, Melanie Klein, pushed aside everything which was in her way, developed her own ideas, had her followers, and built what is in my view a new theory. I think Martin Bergmann made a distinction between extenders and modifiers. Melanie Klein's work was not an extension of Freud's work. It started like this, because when you read the early writings of Melanie Klein, all the time she claims that she is leaning on what Freud had said. But as time went by, she didn't need that any more, and she went her own way – as Lacan did. So these people were not so much quarrelling with Freud, they went forward. To tell you the truth, no one is more critical and lucid about Freud than Freud is himself. But it seems that psychoanalysis reached a dead end. The dead end was: well, here we have this concept of the drives and here we have to admit that we cannot clarify it any further. We lack the intellectual tools to clarify the useful concepts of our theory. When at the end of his life Freud tries to work out what are the impasses in psychoanalytic treatment, he speaks of the dynamic point of view and says, 'When you go beyond the distinction between conscious, pre-conscious, and unconscious, when you want to go deeper, you are sure of ... nothing!' In another paper, he said almost the same thing: in the *Encyclopaedia* paper, Freud wrote that psychoanalysis considered the psychic processes as the result of the interplay of forces which combine themselves and are antagonistic to each other, with all sorts of mixtures, opposition, collaboration. And he says that these forces, which he finds behind the scenes as hypotheses, can be tested in the psychoanalytic treatment either through representations cathected with affects (and here Freud is very clear: what he means is that when you are listening to a patient, what goes on between him and you consists of representations cathected with affects). But if he wants to conceptualise what is the latent structure of what we witness, his answer is that it is the interplay of forces to which he gives the name of drives. He will then, in the text, refer to these forces as belonging to the ego or to sexuality and he will finally give, we are in 1926, the last theory of the drives, the erotic ones and the destructive ones. This is unimportant. The thing that is important is the distinction, which Freud made between what is phenomenologically testable in the analytic situation (with which many people will agree) and the concepts which *he* considers as indispensable to understand it. And here we are obliged to turn to what I was saying earlier: Freud's need to be consistent. For Freud, because of his training, it is impossible to build a theory without a biological background. Some people will totally disagree; they refuse to be constrained by this hypothesis. Nevertheless, when you ask them where does it come from, what are you going to do with the brain, they are very embarrassed and their answers are very poor. The British are clever: they don't bother with the problem. They go forward, not just in any direction; they go forward in a very precise direction. Freud, in the same paper of 1926, after having postulated these drives, says: the most difficult problem the child will have to solve is the Oedipus complex – his relationship to his parents. When you talk about the Oedipus complex, people think, 'aha, yes, we know what he's talking about'. But the British suggested that we can also 'observe' what comes earlier, and therefore – thanks to Melanie Klein – we have now many things happening before the Oedipus complex, 'ah, the Oedipus complex arrives much earlier'. Really! This gives a completely different picture of what it is all about; the father's penis in the mother's womb is not exactly what Freud described, but – the British must have felt – at least there was hope: the relief that one wouldn't be forced to say, 'we don't know ...' Instead, 'Here we have a way, let's focus on children.' It's interesting. In the beginning, it was not a matter of baby observation; it was child psychoanalysis, which of course nobody would object to. Melanie Klein and Anna Freud disagreed, there were lots of discussions. Was it psychoanalysis? Wasn't it psychoanalysis? What was the aim of it? Was it pedagogic? Was it analysis of transference? But in the beginning it was only the extension of psychoanalysis in the direction of the child. And, then, what happened? The extension was not only from the psychoanalysis of the adults to the analysis of the children, but it became the 'knowledge' about the child, 'beyond' psychoanalysis.

There are two ways of considering the child. One way is to include the knowledge of the child into the knowledge of psychoanalysis. Psychoanalysis: you have different sorts – adults, children, psychotics, psychosomatics, delinquents, whatever. But there is another way of including child psychoanalysis. It is to put it in a network of disciplines where you can find paediatrics, child psychiatry, pedagogy, child observation, and so on. What happens then? It happens that the psychoanalytic point of view is drowned and we get child observation occupying the position of a fundamental 'science' in the general theory of child and adult psychoanalysis. We started with Spitz. From Spitz, we went to Mahler. From Mahler, we went all over the place. Am I defending my family, so nobody should come and invade us? No. I'm defending a state of mind. These people are very respectable people, but they do not think as psychoanalysts. We cannot be tricked into thinking that they are going to solve the problems to which we are confronted theoretically. One more word about this: all this happened before, much earlier. With Hartmann, what we saw was the triumph and return of Piaget. In France, we were totally stuck, because, as psychoanalysts, we had spent years and years fighting Piaget's intellectualistic conception, and there it was, all coming back with Hartmann, who believed that that was the type of research that we should have been doing.

GK   In the 1970s, there was an interesting paper by Anne-Marie Sandler linking Piaget with psychoanalysis.[5]

AG   Yes, I told her, that was not right, but Anne-Marie has excuses: she comes from Geneva and was taught by Piaget, but Hartmann didn't need Piaget. The situation is complicated. In reading psychoanalytic literature one has to try to catch what was the spirit of the time, what was the state of mind of that time. Hartmann never gave up the drives, he uses the concept of drives, but his aim was to develop a general psychology. On the one side, he doesn't want to say that he leaves the theory of drives completely behind; on the other hand, of course, this is understandable: you can say drives exist, but there is an autonomous ego, you split the ego from the id, and so that's it, you can build your general psychology. This is not any longer, as far as I am concerned, psychoanalysis: the ego does not come out of a differentiation from the id, it has an origin of its own. Now, I'm not stupid. I do not think that you should believe in the id as something existing, as an entity that can be delineated and proved. But I hardly see what can be 'proved' in psychoanalysis. This idea about the ego of the Ego psychologists is the most natural idea that comes to mind. Why? Because we were never able to give up entirely the conception of the ego as Me, You, the Person, and to emphasise this again and again: in Freud, it is only an instance which can be defined through its relationship to the others. We need a constant reminder of what we are doing, and of what we are thinking, in order not to fall in the trap of academic psychology. I wouldn't say that the French could be characterised as being 'uncompromising' Freudians, but we don't want to go backwards. We don't want to go back to phenomenology; we don't want to go back to psychology. We consider that the Freudian discovery has been a mutation, a radical change of perspectives, and *that* we will keep in mind: what we are trying to talk about is always the subject of the unconscious and that the unconscious's closest links are with wishes, desires, or drives. Now, what does that mean? It means that we will place at the centre of our thinking the idea that, as Freud said, the ego is not master in its own house. And it will never be. It is in that sense that we were all behind Lacan when he opposed Hartmann. If you say that there is an autonomous ego, it means that there is a possibility that the ego would escape the influence of the unconscious, of the drives, and God knows what else.

In discussing the drives, we need to talk about the concept of the object. I wrote a paper to show that there was no possibility of having a unified conception of the object. And this is one of my objections to the Kleinians, because the Kleinians speak of 'the object relationship', meaning that it is the relationship with the first object, the mother, which overshadows everything else. However, is it the breast? Is it the person of the mother? Never mind that anyhow. The important thing is that the father in their view comes *afterwards*! And I say: in their case, the father comes after the curtain has already fallen. The play has been played; the father comes as the second poor chap who is nearly a replica of the mother, with some distinctive traits, oh yes, but of minor importance. We will always agree with them that it is the first relationship, the earliest relationship that is, the most important one. But when you summarise all the different conceptions of the object in Freud, you will find at least five or six opposite conceptions, which are impossible to unify into one. So that led me to make a distinction between – and this does not exist in the English language – between *objective* and *objectal*. In English, you only have 'object relationship', and you only have one word to relate to objectivity or to object relationship. What I have proposed is the concept of what I have called the 'objectalising function'. What I mean is that one of the main aims of psychic function is to create objects. Not only to relate to objects but to create them. This is a simple example: if you take a stamp collector, you're speaking of sublimation; the object is not the stamp, it is the sublimation process. So this is what I mean by objectalising function, the function that Freud describes very well in *The Ego and the Id*, how the ego claims to replace the object. And he imagines this dialogue in which the ego says to the id, 'look, I look so much like the object, you can love me'. So this is an example which shows that Freud understood perfectly well the objectalising process. I think that this is a very important line of thought, the roots of which can be found in identification. Identification is a very special process. Identification is related not to the drive, but to the object.

What is the ego? Is the ego the ego of the businessman who makes good investments, makes a lot of money, controls his agency, and is a successful business man? Why not? Is the ego this organisation which is still bound to the id, whatever it may do? Most of the time, the ego just rationalises, and this is of course a major contribution in Lacan: he showed the rationalisations and illusions that the ego suffers from. The idea of a strong ego, of strengthening the ego -which was so popular in America during the 1950s and 1960s – always appeared to the French as a mystification. But this is still present today. There is a kind of psycho-analytic theory that says, 'Yes, of course, we know we have an uncon-scious, but once we have analysed it, it is under control.' This will kill psychoanalysis in the end. Everything shows – and especially, let's face it, in psychoanalytic circles – that people do not control anything in their unconscious ...

Freud's work is divided in two parts, both clinical. The first part goes till 1924. The metapsychology is a composite book. First paper, 'Instincts and their vicissitudes'. No mention of repression whatsoever. Second paper, 'Repression'. What does it deal with? Not perversion, only neu-rosis. Third paper, 'The unconscious'. What does it deal with? It takes up repression again, it describes the unconscious, and brings in psychosis, considering the relationship between thing- and word-presentation. Fourth paper, the paper on dreams. Hallucination, as a link with the psychoses; the relationship of hallucination with dreams and the question of reality testing. And finally! 'Mourning and melancholia'. So we can see how he started with repression as a model and arrived at the end with mourning and melancholia, shifting from representation to the object. The paper on repression, the paper on the unconscious, and even the paper on dreams are all focused on representations and perceptions, but with 'Mourning and melancholia', it is on the object and cathexis, the object and the replacement of the lost object by part of the ego.

It is very important that from 1924 onwards, Freud changes his model. The relationship is not any more between neurosis and perversion; it is be-tween neurosis and psychosis. Other points are points of articulation, for example, fetishism. Why? Because it's still perversion but he is describing a splitting, a mechanism which will be extended to psychosis in *The Outline* ... It is very important to make this distinction; Freud is an-nouncing to us the development of borderline phenomena. If you read Freud carefully, there are many indications of the persistence of normal life in psychosis; he would say, for instance, that in psychosis we may have an ego which crumbles, which is completely broken down, though a normal perception still goes on in some corners of the mind. In other cases, we can have cases in which the ego's unity is compromised, the ego splits itself. The follies of man are to the ego what perversions are to sexuality. My God, how can people have read Freud so many times and completely ignore such an important remark? It was obvious that in the end of his life he foresaw that the future of therapeutic analysis would have to deal with this structure. Of course, he had no idea of Klein ...

GK Again, French psychoanalysis seemed to have moved in a different way to almost the rest of the world: while still considering and treating borderline phenomena, you didn't abandon the neuroses.

AG In the Anglo-Saxon model, the basic hypothesis is the hierarchy. The earlier, the deeper.

GK I agree. That's a point I have always argued against.

AG If one makes progress in analytic knowledge, one is supposed to get closer and closer to the original psychosis. Even if you didn't call it that. The Americans will not agree with the term 'original psychosis' but oh! the Americans are so very excited because they have now discovered pre-genitality. They will say, 'Oedipus is nothing, pre-genitality is all.' I am trying to fight for something quite different. The analyst needs to work with different models. One model does not replace another model because it is earlier or it is more regressive. I have to think with the neurosis model, with the borderline model, according to each patient. And it may happen that in different moments of the same analysis I will have to shift from one model to another. In borderlines, the resistance to change is considerable, but maybe I will use here Balint's expression, 'a limited change, though of considerable importance'. I will make a distinction between two types of borderline. Because, you know, it is impossible now to continue to talk of borderline, because borderline is not an entity, it's a continent! Today I think of borderline patients, less in terms of them standing on a border between neurosis and psychosis (although this is indeed the situation in many of them) but more as these people living in a sort of no man's land, turning round and round some roundabout from which they can take many directions without engaging themselves in any one of them (depression, perversion, character disorder, or even psychosomatic conditions). When you say 'borderline', one can oppose it to almost everything. There are two types of borderline for me: those who after years of treatment I shall feel able to put on the couch, and those for which this can never happen, and this is a clinical difference. Who of the two is the most ill? Boundaries and issues are completely blurred by external criteria: they work, they don't work. Now, most of my very ill borderline patients are psychiatrists. The findings of Winnicott and of Bion are of utmost importance in this area. That is why I admire them. I admire them because I feel at home when I read them; I understand what they say. But some analysts in France - I don't know if this is the case in England – say that they can't read Bion for more than two pages, the book falls from their hands. I say to them, 'Well, I'm sorry for you because I think the knowledge contained in his writings is essential.'

GK   Bion is very well respected in England, and in Latin America, although I'm not so sure that he is understood.

AG   This is another question. That applies to other authors too. As I said to David Tuckett once, 'your Winnicott is not our Winnicott'.

GK   Now, to go back a bit. I've raised the question of the institution ...

AG   I think it's time to talk about that. I think that, unfortunately, analytic institutions are in a very difficult position now. They have played with denial, 'business as usual', everybody felt that something was wrong, but nobody has done anything about it. I am not going to go into the training procedures, by-laws and regulations and so on, I'm not interested in that. Recently, I was invited to take part in a meeting in New York. The meeting was about the evaluation of the Hartmann era. There were seven or eight people who were invited. There were only two foreigners, Clifford Yorke, from London, and myself, the rest of them were American; we discussed and argued for two days. We started with a paper by Martin Bergmann, a huge paper, 80 pages, very well researched, and each of us discussed the paper and gave a contribution, and so on. In the end, the final summary was very critical of Hartmann, and critical of the Hartmannites – as Bergmann calls them – and I said to these gentlemen, 'Look, what you are proving is that the International Congresses are totally useless.' Their protest against the Hartmann era is recent, maybe five years ago. So I said, 'May I remind you that Winnicott's paper on the metapsychological and clinical use of regression is dated 1954! May I remind you that until that time, we have been from one congress to another, listening to endless debates between opposite points of views, and this means that after each congress everyone went back home, forgetting everything that had been said. You became amnesiac and you became deaf, what's the use of congresses?' Did you know that American analysts were not allowed to read Melanie Klein? In their institutes, there was no teaching of Melanie Klein. I do not know for sure, but it is obvious that Hartmann was taught in London, even though nobody paid much attention to him, not even Anna Freud. Institutions fail in their task of raising questions of real interest and debate. Science becomes political; institutes are institutions in which the people who hold the power try to promote their own theory, or at least do not give a chance of hearing theories which run against them. Unless we do something about it, psychoanalysis is going to die from the inside, not from the attacks of the outside. When I discussed Jacobs' paper in Amsterdam, there was a lot of turmoil and upset because I really, truly wanted to discuss it. Jacobs didn't say hello to me for six months; I was insulted during the intervals. Only my British friends came to me and were supportive. Theory is so grounded in the narcissism of the analyst that people do not dare to have any discussion. I believe that there is a difference with the French, because we had to learn being attacked by the Lacanians and had no other choice than to reply, which meant that we had to read, to think, to argue ...

GK   In spite of your pessimism about the scientific life of psychoanalytic institutions, you very actively participate in them. Do you think we need psychoanalytic societies?

AG   You would be very popular in France if you were to say that, because people have raised the question, 'Why do we have to be part of an institution who only asks us for very high fees and give us what in return?'

GK   You were saying more, you were suggesting that psychoanalysis is being killed by the institution. Now, that is a serious statement.

AG   Yes, yes, what I say is two statements. The first one is: psychoanalysis will never be accepted by the culture. Never!

GK   That shouldn't worry us so much. Psychoanalysis, by definition, cannot be accepted by the culture. Something in psychoanalysis is killed whenever it is accepted by society.

AG   Agreed. Today we have enough evidence to show that when the culture pretends to accept it, it's only when it is presented with a view of psychoanalysis which fits its own requirements. This didn't happen in America only. In France, Lacan himself was also another example. People were amused by Lacan for 10 years, and after 10 years he vanished, disappeared, sunk without trace. From the cultural point of view we have nothing to hope for. We cannot be accepted by society, we will never have a seat at the various Academies. From within, the killing of psychoanalysis is due to the bureaucracy and the struggle for power, which is also ideological. There is a kind of consensus that we should accept to discuss things with everyone but, in fact, people feel very threatened if you open the discussion widely. In part, I think this is because of the nature of psychoanalytic practice. You stay all day in your armchair; you cannot reply; you are loved and cherished or hated and abused, but you know it's not for yourself ... You cannot use the ordinary means of trying to convince people that this thing works; it's really a burden, a terrible burden. It is then normal that the institution is the reservoir of all, I wouldn't call 'the psychotic anxieties', I'm not interested in that, but I'm interested in the narcissistic side, the narcissistic safeguard of the analyst. Let's think of ourselves as cardiologists. If you want to defend an idea about how a disease comes about and someone comes after you and says, 'No, Dr Kohon, you're not right, I have statistical evidence to show it, and here is the best theory to explain that. It's painful but it's life!' In analysis, if I say my theory is better than yours is, it means that you are stupid, or ill, or both! Or that you haven't been properly analysed. This is too much. This is why we have the most awful thing that can happen to an analytic society: militantism. I am very proud to belong to a society, the Paris Society, which has no militants. We have no Kleinians; we have no Kohutians; we have no ego–psychologists, and we have, let's say, half a dozen theoreticians who have their own ideas. People make up their minds by debating, by going to them, listening to them, working with them.

GK You recently told me about your decision not to accept to be a candidate for the International's presidency ...

AG My God!

GK Let's imagine that you had decided for a positive decision, and that you would have been elected. Obviously, there was a project in mind; you would have wanted to carry out this project. What do you think you would have wanted to do? You had a vision; what did it consist of?

AG My relationship with the International developed in two periods. The first period was from 1973 to 1977 and the second period started in 1989. The explanation of this gap is the following. In Paris, 1973, I was a member of the programme committee after the Vienna Congress of 1971. I had had a bad experience in 1973. I should not develop this point; there were too many political games being played out then. I considered running for the vice-presidency. I was standing from the floor and there were people who supported me, but there had also been very strong pressure from the Executive, headed by Rangell at the time and under the influence of Lebovici insisting that I should withdraw. Finally, I did withdraw. I didn't want to take advantage that the Congress, being in Paris, the assembly would have elected me. Anyhow, some people were very kind to me, especially the British, who then supported me in London in 1975 when I was indeed elected. The important thing is that in 1977 I decided to withdraw from all administrative business and to devote myself to scientific tasks. Also, at the time I had to settle very important personal problems and I had to restrict my time. I said that I didn't want to do any administrative work, but I was still ready to co-operate scientifically whenever I was needed. But I was left aside completely from 1977 to 1989, even for scientific contributions. What are the reasons for that? To run for president was not in my mind at all at that time, but some people preferred to leave me aside; they feared that I would become popular and would run, and as there was a next European presidency, I could be the person to stir things up. It was only after Joe Sandler was elected that I was invited once again to participate in the scientific programmes, as another European President would have only been elected twelve years later. I was interested in scientific work, not to stand on committees to sort the problem of a split in a Society here or there, or to improve the constitutional by-laws, or anything of the kind. For that, I have no personal inclination.

Meanwhile, after having settled the problems in my private life, in 1986 I became president of the Paris Society. Everyone remembers this period of my presidency as having brought a *renaissance* in the Society on many grounds. I accepted to run as president of the Paris Society only when the statutes had been changed and voted for, otherwise I would have been president much earlier. I had been asked many times before, but I refused because I thought that the statutes were inappropriate, created tensions and difficulties, and I didn't want to participate in a structure which I knew was not workable. So when the statutes were changed, I applied. If I had not taken this break in 1977, I would have run in due time, but I had more urgent things to do. Then, when Horacio Etchegoyen was appointed as president, he and the people around him really wanted me to run this time. I considered the situation for two years, thinking what I would do, what was possible to do and so on. In the end, I decided to abstain. And so, now we come to your question, what would I have done? I have given a lot of thought to it. There are three problems, all closely linked with each other: the shortage of patients, the loss of prestige of psychoanalysis, and the division amongst the psychoanalysts. One of the most important problems is that psychoanalysts are out of touch with what other disciplines are saying. My vision would have been the following: first, my priority would have been to try to restore some trust in psychoanalytic practice. Now, I know from our conversations that you do not think that the crisis has only negative aspects, that there are also positive aspects. I understand what you mean; I am not the kind of person who thinks that the more psychoanalysts we have the better it will be – this is not at all my feeling. I am rather an elitist; I would prefer maybe fewer of us and more psychoanalytically trained people with a rigorous mind who discuss things in depth. I am not at all for the extension of psychoanalysis in all directions. I do not think psychoanalysis can die, but I think it will lose twenty-five years. It may take that many years before people realise what illusions they have invested in the neuro-sciences or chemical treatments, and so on, and they will come back to psychoanalysis, and when they come back to it, psychoanalysis will not be the same, it will have changed. So if we can avoid losing these twenty-five years, I think we should start immediately. How? I would say there are two fronts: foreign policies and internal policies. The foreign policies: since 1953, when I was a psychiatrist, I have always heard that psychoanalysis would die the following year. All sorts of reasons and pretexts were given to sustain this opinion. 1953 was the year I started my psychiatric training; it was also the year when psychotropic drugs were invented. People believed that with the drugs, 'no problems, everything would be cured, no need for psychoanalysis any more'. After that, we had many other attacks. We were attacked by the Marxists, an attack which was very strong even earlier. We then had the attacks by the structuralist movement. Endlessly, endlessly. The great news was that psychoanalysis was dying: if not now, it will be dead next year. The difference is that this time, contemporary attacks come from the new sciences of the brain. Now, I do not think that because they come from neuro-sciences they are more serious, but people can be more impressed. The attitude of psychoanalysts was, for a long time, the one that recommended, 'ignore the criticism and go on'. This time you cannot afford it. In the past, science had nothing to offer; it's different now. We have to respond to these attacks.

GK You know, this makes me think of something completely different, but you'll see the point in the end. You must have known, or have heard of Enrique Pichon-Riviére.

AG Yes, of course.

GK He was asked once to conduct an investigation into the Jewish community in Buenos Aires, which had been under a series of attacks – synagogues, cultural centres, etc. There was always a strong involvement of the analysts in Argentina with institutional work, with social psychology. The question was, why, at that particular historical moment, there had been such a widespread series of attacks? Was there something to be said about the Jewish community itself that was – not provoking the attacks – but facilitating them? A part of the conclusion was, in fact, that the Jewish community was very divided; their internal divisions were such that it was just possible that they were offering themselves as victims. The neo-Nazis were simply exploiting the cracks within the Jewish community. I know, this is very controversial, and very, very simplified. But is there something similar to be said about the psychoanalytic community? Are our own internal divisions, disagreements, confusions, and insecurities – are they facilitating the attacks from the enemies of psychoanalysis?

AG Oh, yes, of course.

GK Should we concentrate on our own internal affairs, more than on the outsiders' attacks? Is the main problem the lack of belief in psychoanalysis, the disappointments, and the lack of conviction of the analysts themselves?

AG We have to worry about both, inside and outside. We have been attacked by the neuro-biologists and specialists of the brain, and this is the thing that we have to keep in mind. The closer people are to what we do, the brain and the mind or the body–mind problem, the more they fiercely attack us. This is not a problem of 'objective knowledge'; this is a subjective problem of inner beliefs, of prejudice, of refusing to take into account some things that we think are very important and cannot be ignored. Today, it is the progress of the neuro-scientist, the brain specialist, which is the most harmful to us. On the contrary, as far as I have experienced it, those who deal with general biology are sympathetic to us. I can give names, but I will only mention one – Gerald Edelman. But he is not a specialist of brain mechanisms, he's an immunologist who turned to the study of the brain afterwards and wrote these important books on consciousness, one of them being dedicated to Darwin and Freud.[6] So it is not that we have everybody against us. Now, what you say about psychoanalysts ... I tell you, it's even much worse. Psychoanalysts are careless. As long as they have their practice filled, and it's not very difficult to fill it with other psychoanalysts, they don't care. They only started to worry because of the shortage of patients. I think we urgently have to come back into the debate, and we have to organise meetings to talk with these people. But this means that psychoanalysts must know what these people do: what are their writings? What are their own concerns? What are their methods? What are the limitations in what they find? This needs a lot of work. We are in a situation of war. Unless we do it, I am sure that we are going to have a very bad time. This, I would say, is the foreign policy. It is very interesting, for instance, when you listen to what Otto Kernberg says about the situation in the previous generation, between the people who had been appointed at the university as Professors of Psychiatry, and the people who remained in the institutions as training analysts in the USA. In fact, these two parties fought separately, one ignoring the other, instead of uniting their efforts. And I think that nowadays we have to ensure a presence in the institutions that treat patients. If psychoanalysts work in these institutions, if they can show the residents, for example, the medical students, the difference between a patient who is seen by an analyst and the same patient seen by a non-analyst, it is obvious that the situation will return to our advantage. This will not be easy because they don't want us to be back in the institutions.

The second thing, the internal affairs, and the division amongst psychoanalysts: this is a dreadful problem. We need to find ways and take the time to ask very serious questions to our colleagues: why do you say this? On what grounds? What are the clinical implications? What are the technical consequences? Of course, I'm not that naïve to the point of thinking that a general reconciliation will emerge from all that, but at least we will be able to clarify our differences, the disagreements between the different families of psychoanalysis today, and maybe that will help. I do not believe that psychoanalytic congresses can fulfil that function. Instead, I believe that, let's say, the leaders of theoretical thought should have the possibility of meeting regularly, taking time not only to expose what we already know, but also to really discuss and clarify our ideas about what we do not know. I think this is very important, to try to explain the historical revolution that happened in such a country that led to this and that theory. Why was it thought to be better than what was there earlier, or what was done on the other side of the ocean, and so on? I believe that these in-depth theoretical exchanges between analysts might help. It will take time but at least it may bring some change. France is a very good example. We had a very hard time with Lacan. Lacan was not like Melanie Klein; Melanie Klein remained in the Society; the Kleinians were present, and every group examined their ideas, but you were still in the same space and you still had meetings in which different points of view were expressed. Lacan was attacking us fiercely from outside. There had been two tactics to deal with this. One proved to be a disaster – ignoring what he said. It was believed that the less you talked about Lacan, the better it would be. It failed. The second tactic, which is the example of my generation, was to say, 'Let's go and see what he has to offer.' I spent six years going to Lacan's seminars, having permanent discussions with him, and finally, I knew something about what he said. If I disagreed with him, it was from a position of knowledge. I could do it. One thing, which is very important, is the question of one generation after another. The generation of my elders was involved in personal quarrels that were not mine. Nacht, Lacan, Lebovici, Lagache. For us, it wasn't important, but we still had an attitude of combat. Maybe we had lost the historical development, but at least we could read the text with an open mind, and make our own minds up without being involved in personal quarrels. An open mind is essential. For many years, in the 1960s, Klein was really the devil in America. Look at it now: you see quite a number of people coming up with interesting ideas, often having obviously been influenced by the British school. You could not imagine Ogden, who is a very respectable person and who has developed an interesting perspective in psychoanalysis, you couldn't imagine him without the influence of the British school. So, a proper exchange of ideas would definitely help. But, one has to say, Ogden is not part of the institutional system; he remains on his own.

GK   There is a certain irony in the fact that while psychoanalysis has been suffering so many attacks, it has also greatly influenced the academic world, both in the USA and in England. There have been intense de-bates, theoretical exchanges, and interesting ideas developing *outside* the Societies.

AG   Of course, I agree. For Freud, this was evident. Applied psychoanalysis is important. Some of his works of applied psychoanalysis were based on an error, but still, they were addressing very important issues. Can you ignore the *Leonardo* in the art history departments? After Freud, psycho-analysts not only committed errors; they were also superficial in these attempts. They gave up, and this task has been taken up by other people, who might write very important and interesting things. Within the psychoanalytic movement, psychoanalytic theory has been reduced to the theory of the cure, which I think is terribly harmful. Firstly, it doesn't solve anything, and secondly, it leads to over-simplifications. In many psychoanalytic circles one of the consequences has been the theoretical over-use of object relations theory. Because, if you consider that analysis is essentially the theory of what happens during the analytic cure, then all you have is object relations theory. These people do not seem to worry at all about what happens to the baby when he is not with the mother. What goes on in his mind? How has his relationship been transformed when he is alone? In other words, what's going on in the intra-psychic world? It is impossible just to consider psychoanalytic theory as the result of psychoanalytic cure. Of course, the British are really the people who have extended our clinical experience: they have taken risks. We owe it to Melanie Klein, to the Kleinians, to Bion and Winnicott, and I would say to most of the people of the British school, we owe to them the extension of the frontiers of psychoanalysis. The question which arises here is, if you are a purist, is this still psychoanalysis? We know that serious objections can be made to Winnicott's work, and Winnicott himself did not hide it. He said, 'When I can do psychoanalysis, I do psychoanalysis; when I can't do it then, I do what I can.' What he did, no one who was *not* a psychoanalyst could have done it … and it could not be labelled as 'psychotherapy'! So I think that it is very important for us to be aware that the richness of psychoanalysis is due to the extension of the field. But how do we arrive at an agreement with no exclusions?

GK   Talking about applied psychoanalysis, there is something else in all this. If we take as an example, let's say, *Totem and Taboo*, the whole book is based on the wrong anthropological assumptions, and yet the questions that Freud has brought up in that text have not been answered or re-solved. He made mistakes, but what great mistakes they were! There seems to be, at the basis of the disagreements about texts like *Totem and Taboo*, different theoretical understandings about the structure of the unconscious, or maybe to put it more precisely, about the understanding of the unconscious *as structure*.

AG   It is true. I have to say two things about what you say. I am old enough to have seen many different periods in the relationship between psycho-analysis and other disciplines. For instance the relationship with anthro-pology. For nearly twenty-five years, at least, even more, even thirty years, it was impossible for an analyst (if one was not on the side of Lacan leaning on Lévi-Strauss) to say anything about anthropology. One would be attacked, considered as old hat, or whatever. But nothing is eternal. Last June (1997), we had a meeting in which there were anthropologists and psychoanalysts discussing many different issues. There was openness about new ideas. The question was, 'Is psychoanalytic anthropology possible?' I have been now working for four years with one anthropolo-gist. So things change. You speak of structure. You are obviously pin-pointing a very important issue. The reason why people in England are struck by such an issue is that they only know one conception of the unconscious: the historic one. The baby, from birth to adulthood.

Whether you call it development, or maturational process, it's always the same thing. It was Lacan who really taught us that this perspective could lead to very wrong ideas precisely because of all the excesses of the so-called genetic point of view. But here we have another problem, because Lacan went in the direction of structuralism. Structuralism is a point of view which goes against the historical one: the whole thing is thought out in Lacan from a linguistic Saussurian point of view. Before Saussure, people were almost entirely interested in etymology, where did the words come from? What transformations had occurred? With Saussure came the idea that the relationship between the terms was more important than the relationship of a term to its meaning. But in my opinion, Lacan failed. He said, 'the unconscious is structured like a language'. But even if you do not agree with him that the unconscious is structured like a language, and you consider that the structure of the unconscious is different from the structure of language, what remains is the idea of structure. There are two meanings of structure that are contradictory. One, which is the old, more traditional one, is equated with architecture. For instance, you've studied Henry Ey. His point of view was that structure was the 'architecture' of what we are supposed to find at the bottom of the causality of mental illness. But there is another, different meaning: structure as this network of relationships which are not hierarchically built, but with a special organisation at each different level. We can see the applications very easily. For instance, let us take a very simple matter, the structure of the pre-conscious. In the pre-conscious you have words and thoughts, but in the unconscious you are not supposed to have words and thoughts, you only have thing-presentations. This is something that for us is very important, but the British never use it – what Freud calls the attraction in the already repressed; when something is repressed it doesn't get lost or isolated; it is called by something which is *already structured*. The structural point of view, in this context, can only be understood in terms of a conflict of structures. There are always two sources, a double polarity: what comes from the biological, and what comes from society, history, and tradition. We understand nowadays that structure is an absolutely necessary concept; an ontogenetic point of view will never give us the clues for our psychoanalytic understanding. Let me give you an example, because I think it is important. There is a concept in psychoanalysis which is rejected unanimously by psychoanalysts: primal fantasies.

GK   Most analysts would reject them.

AG   Yes, well, primal fantasy would be rejected by science too. What can one say about primal fantasies? How do you account for the fact that, in every individual life, there is a variety of experiences, which are so many, all kinds of experiences happen to different people, but they seem to be organised according to a set of parameters of phantasy? Lacan gave them a good name: 'key signifiers'. Whatever you call them, key signifiers or primal fantasies, the idea is the same: something has to regulate this multiplicity of experiences, a small set of regulators which puts order to the chaos of experience. I differ from Freud. For instance, he said that these primal fantasies 'corrected' the happenings that were 'too individual'. For instance, he would say that, in the Wolf Man, there is a submission to the father, a homosexual one – but the father would remain the castrator in his elaboration. So for him, the function of the father as the castrator superseded this individual conjuncture, this particular circumstance, in which the boy submitted to the father instead of opposing him. I differ from Freud because I think again we must be able to work with two or three constellations. He wanted a unifying Oedipus complex; everything had to converge there. I think that we can now work with different models: the model of neurosis, the borderline model, the model of psychosomatics, etc. There are other constellations, for example, the constellation in which the mother is dominant or omnipotent, or the one in which the father is dominant, and maybe a third one, with different variations. And then in the analysis we have to play with that. With different patients, one model seems to apply better than others.

GK   What remains difficult to understand is that the external events, the mother or the father or whatever, are not determining the structure; it's something that comes *with* the structure. Castration, the primal scene, these come 'with' the structure, they are part and parcel of the structure.

AG   Oh yes, of course.

GK   You say 'of course' ...

AG   When I say of course, I mean, this needs an explanation.

GK   Most people seem to talk about these issues in very naturalistic ways.

AG   Yes, that is the point. Let us take a very simple example because everyone has it in mind: the Oedipus complex. Let's consider for a moment Lacan's argument. Lacan says it is nonsensical to speak of pre-Oedipal stages. You can speak of pre-genital phases, but not pre-Oedipal. Why? Lacan emphasises something that is absolutely self-evident and undebatable: that when the child arrives in the world, he is already structured by the Oedipal conflict of its parents. So before even the child experiences the first smile, the mother has already a complete programme of fantasies, and the father too; there is a relationship between the three players in this drama ... even before the baby was born. So it is impossible to speak of this phase as being 'pre-Oedipal'. Let us take now the Oedipal situation *per se*. I wonder if the British have ever read the two pages, which Freud devoted to it, because he only devoted two pages. He first described it in 1897, then forgot it, and brought it back, out of the blue, in 1923. My God, what did he do before 1923? He wrote *Totem and Taboo*. What was the idea? Freud did not want to give an individual interpretation of Oedipus. He had first to link it to culture, then he had to theorise the superego, and only then he could describe what happened to the individual. Now, in these two pages, what does he say? First, he describes a general structure and in the general structure he describes the positive Oedipus complex and then the negative complex, and he says that in every case we only have bits which survive from the positive and from the negative. So we don't have a triangle, we have a lozenge, with the positive and the negative. I would say, using another vocabulary, that one is dominant and the other is recessive and when the recessive becomes dominant (the cases when there is a negative Oedipus complex), we know we are going to have much more trouble. Let's take the simplest, the positive Oedipus complex with the male boy. Positive relationship to the mother, which is labelled in terms of desire, and on the other side, the father, the child's identification with his father, the hostility leading to identification. Let us take now the negative one – it's exactly the reverse: desire for the father, identification with the mother. And so now we understand that *desire* and *identification* are here parts of the structure, complementary, opposite, and symmetrical. There is a very strong link within desire and identification, which is not clarified. Where is the clarification? If you read Freud carefully, you see that the clarification is that desire has always to do with contact, as when Freud says the relationship of the child to the breast is one of the most important ones, and it is the prototype of all future loving relationships. When he speaks of identification with the father, what is he talking about? He speaks of the identification with what he calls the father of the pre-history. He says that in the beginning, the child has absolutely no feeling of rivalry toward the father, all he wants is to be like him. Here, there is no contact, only admiration in a distant relationship. Now, of course you can say, 'but what about the situation in which it is the reverse?' It cannot be the reverse. Why? Because the father hasn't borne the child nine months in his belly. The contact between the mother and the child is always, always different to the contact that the child will have with the father. If you consider nowadays the new parents, the contemporary fathers who are feeding, giving the bottle to the babies, etc., what do we see? That to the eyes of the mother, the father is always incompetent. He can pretend to know what to do, but only the mother really knows it. The idea of structure does not only describe something which happens at a certain stage, but it creates the possibility of understanding the internal contradictions of a situation of which you will have, in the analytic session, only bits of the two different Oedipal dilemmas, the positive and the negative, and it's up to the analyst to reconstitute the whole thing. When we come to the primal fantasies also, what we have here is a setting. The primal fantasies have been described by Freud as seduction, castration, primal scene. But if you think of them not only as a list of items, you see that there is a consistency. Seduction leads to castration: you have to be punished for the pleasure that you inappropriately had. Castration will define your position in the primal scene, the seduction relationship of two others who exclude the subject, whether you identify with the one who bears the phallus, or with the one who is submitted to the power of the phallus. When one takes this to the analyst in the situation of treatment, one realises that it's all a question of the analyst's *disposition d'esprit*, the state of mind in which the analyst will be listening to the patient. When a patient says something to me, I will never, never, ever think, 'What age is he talking about? When did this happen? What happened to him at that time?' How could I know? I don't know; I have no possibility of knowing. All I have is the possibility of listening while trying to organise the picture in my mind of what is happening now. Not that we are for the *here and now*; we think that the here and now interpretations may be misleading; the analysis of the patient in the session always refers to *ailleurs, un autre fois*, somewhere else, in another time, some other scene which is not happening in the session.

GK   Do you ever make interpretations in the transference?

AG   Of course I do, all the time, but this is not systematic. I described something which I called the interpretative process. When you are with a borderline patient, for example, I believe it is traumatic for him to receive interpretations. What you offer is an interpretative process. I take what he says and analyse it on a level which is more or less superficial, close to what the patient says. Then, he might say something else and one goes a bit further and then further still; only later one might give a transference interpretation. It is important not to knock the patient with an interpretation but to enable the process to proceed, to enrich itself, to become more and more complex, so when you give the transference interpretation, the patient may experience the value of it. He can understand that it refers to something here and now, between you and himself, and also to what happens outside with his girlfriend, to what we have been saying about his relationship with his brother, father or whoever long ago. An interpretation spreads on many levels and diverse feelings and different situations and can refer to what has been said earlier on in another session, and this is only possible if you are free *not* to think in terms of babies; in your interpretation you can have all the same, the baby, the 3-year-old child, the adolescent, and even the old man that he is not yet. And this is only possible because there is a structure.

GK   You talk in terms of a *disposition d'esprit*. This state of mind depends on how the analyst sees and experiences his own position in relation to his patient, and how he sees and experiences the patient. Sometimes, some analysts seem to start making interpretations in the transference to the patient, without even considering whether there is a subject there in the first place. The patient then is not treated as an adult, but he is infantilised, or dismissed. On the other hand, I find that it might be necessary to make transference interpretations so the patient could realise, take notice, that there is an other's subjectivity in the room. I believe that one has to offer oneself as an object of transference through these interpretations, which enables the patient to start relating to the analyst; otherwise, sometimes he might just go on talking to himself inside his autistic, neurotic bubble, instead of to me.

AG   How to know that there is a subject? *There will be a subject when a patient tells you a dream.* Then you know that he is a subject. You have associations; the dream unfolds; you have the latent thoughts; you have the fantasy, and so on. If a patient comes and says, 'I want to succeed in my examination; I'm working hard', etc., he doesn't tell you anything. He doesn't tell you if, in fact, he wants to fail which might be the most important piece of information. If you then make an interpretation, saying something about the here and now, you will be automatically transforming the patient into a child. This, the British don't understand. I wrote a paper in 1979 saying that psychoanalysis was now at a crossroads: it was either the child, or the dream. The 'child' represents all this developmental point of view, the misunderstandings created by baby observation and what not. The 'dream' is the true paradigm of psychoanalysis. If Freud had to save one thing, and only one, it would be the dream. It wouldn't be *The Three Essays* ...; the dream develops outside consciousness, it is a true unconscious event. There's the diminution of censorship, and therefore there's the emergence of desire. Bion was the only Kleinian analyst who preferred the dream to the child. And amongst the Independents, Winnicott plainly, explicitly says that the important moment in the therapeutic consultation with a child is the moment when the child is ready to tell a dream.

GK   Sometimes, it seems difficult for many to understand the connection between theory and practice. Many analysts devalue the pursuit of theory, as if it is not very relevant. Psychoanalysis, at one end of the spectrum, seems to have become for many a problem of technique; they are technicians learning a trade. Now, the connection between theory and technique is very close; if one changes the theory, it is inevitable for the technique to change too. For Melanie Klein, for example, the foundation of the subject takes place at the moment of weaning. The separation from the breast is the crucial moment in the constitution of subjectivity. If one believes that this is the most important thing in one's life, then inevitably one would start interpreting separation at the weekends, the anxieties about the holiday breaks, etc. There is never any mention in the cases presented by some colleagues about the possible pleasure a patient might experience in having a holiday. I even find patients who become 'disappointed' when they realise that I don't interpret the separation from the beginning, because they have heard that *that* is what a 'real' analysis is all about.

AG   I think you are right. There is some irony in what you say because, for Melanie Klein, the loss of the object – as the French understand it – does not exist. Freud stated quite clearly that for the reality principle to exist, the object which once provided satisfaction has to be lost. This is totally ignored by Melanie Klein; she wouldn't know what he was referring to. What is the importance of that? The importance is the next statement in Freud: that according to the reality principle, the important event is not to find the object but to re-find it. This dialectic is completely lost in Melanie Klein and all the Kleinians. Winnicott plays with the idea, but he gives an equivalent description. He says: first, we have the subjective object, and then we have the object of perception; this is a paradox for him, which we cannot solve and should not be solved. The subjective object offers the possibility of experiencing the omnipotence and the illusion, and in this way, the continuity between the self and the object. With the perceived object, the subject develops the awareness that the object is separate, that omnipotence doesn't work, that the object is outside and has an independent existence. Winnicott, who seems to have ignored Freud, has kept Freud's structure. In Melanie Klein, the structure is lost, it is nonsensical, it is ignored. I have a couple of friends who follow my ideas very closely; they have summarised this situation in a very beautiful and condensed way. They said: *only inside, also outside.* Only inside is the subjective object, the fantasised object, the object of omnipotence. But if you want to know if it exists or not, you have to check also outside. Only inside, also outside.

GK   The paper on the dead mother has been a very important paper. It's an incredibly difficult paper; it's not an easy paper at all and yet it has had great influence. It is very rich, and there are many levels to it. It goes without saying that there are also many questions to be asked, to be sorted out. Now, I always think that one writes for somebody, perhaps *against* somebody, or a mixture of both.

AG   Yes, you can say that.

GK   Who was in your mind when you wrote that paper?

AG   Firstly, it is true that this paper is the most successful one that I have ever written. I wasn't aware at all that it had been so well received everywhere until I started to see patients in consultations who would come in and start describing the dead mother syndrome to me. In general I am a bit suspicious when people come to me and say things like that. When I think retrospectively about the paper, I think that there is a very interesting combination. The interesting combination is the confluence of a personal experience while I was having my third analysis, of my own clinical experience with patients, and, finally, a theoretical experience. This last one was represented by the impact of Winnicott's paper on transitional objects. Of course, I had been a great admirer and a reader of Winnicott, but it was only when I wrote the paper for the conference in

Milan [included in this volume] that I realised how much the concept of
the transitional object had influenced me, even if I wasn't aware precisely
how it had had this effect. The interesting thing is that when I wrote
'The dead mother' I was not fully aware of what I was saying. You
know, I never write a clinical paper according to the British model:
introduction, the point that you are going to discuss, two pages of bibliography, the clinical material, the discussion of the clinical material,
conclusion, etc. I rarely base a paper on just one patient. When I write a
paper I think of several patients who I believe have something that fits in
with the problem I am dealing with, even if they are very different patients.

GK   One of the things that fascinated me about the paper, something that
immediately resonated within me and my clinical experience, was the
connection between the dead mother syndrome, the notion of a 'patched
breast', and creativity in a number of creative artists, some of whom are
genuinely creative but totally incapable of love.

AG   I had a very narcissistic patient; all of his life he had to carry the burden
of a mother who was supposed not to love the father, who was a good
man but who was also very anxious, highly neurotic, spending hours
praying and praying for the child. The mother had come from a foreign
country; she was very, very proud, and had lost – before the birth of my
patient – a girl who was totally idealised as dead children usually are. All
his life this patient was confronted with his own achievements and the
comparison with this dead girl who was supposed to have been perfect
on all grounds. It was obvious. It appeared to me that the boy was very
lonely and depressed and terribly anxious, with true paranoid anxiety. At
the same time, he had a compulsion to play. He played alone, all the
time. I was a very young analyst then. I thought this was because of his
capacity and his need to fantasise. Finally, I understood that with this
play, he was trying to distract the mother even when he was playing
alone; he was trying to amuse the mother, to get the mother out of her
depression and isolation, trying to get her to leave this idealised young
daughter. In spite of an improvement, I could never really cure him. It
would be too long to tell the entire story. The main problem was that
this is a man who never worked in his life, but he was clever, clever
enough to be supported by his wife's family. He decided to start writing,
and he succeeded! He published some poems in journals of poetry, of a
very high standard. He even started moving around the literary world
and established relationships with well-recognised people in the field.
And then, he stopped. He couldn't go on. We have no time to give the
details of his cyclical structure; we have no time for that. But in the end
he left me, saying, 'Dr Green, in spite of your great efforts, which I
praise, you have not succeeded in detaching me from my mother – you

are just like my father. The bond between my mother and myself is too strong and it is impossible to undo.'

GK   Such grandiosity ...

AG   Yes, but what I wanted to emphasise was the inability to love of some creative people. This man couldn't love anybody. He was married to a young lady who, I think, loved him, but people thought that she was stupid; they despised her. He had affairs with other women, but these women were not important. Then this lady died, accidentally. What happened was extraordinary. The man changed completely. He entirely re-wrote his past, worshipped her, declared how perfect she had been, how much he loved her, he could not live with anyone else, and so on.

GK   Everybody idealises the person they have lost, but you seem to suggest something else: that this patient developed what you call a 'mad passion' for a mother.

AG   Absolutely. He became identified with his own mother mourning her lost daughter. In fact, he did not mourn her, because he would have become aware of how cruel he had been; paradoxically, he got rid of her through idealisation; when alive, he had felt imprisoned by her.

GK   So it was the actualisation of his mad passion for the mother. You talk about this in your paper. I have had the privilege of analysing a number of creative artists and writers, and I also found this contrast between their capacity to create and their incapacity to love; there is an extraordinary moment in the analysis, something absolutely moving, when they are capable of creating or discovering a 'patched' breast, an original object which sustains them.

AG   The result is that any benefit, which comes out of analysis, will go to their art. They will write poetry but they will not change.

GK   This is quite a different conception to the Kleinian understanding of creativity as reparation. Also, in reading 'The dead mother', one understands that you're struggling to make sense of this mad passion for the mother within an Oedipal constellation, but the mad passion for the mother does not include the mother at all. It only includes the unknown object of bereavement, which can be the text created, or the painting, or the piece of music.

AG   Yes, yes.

GK   The third term turns into a peculiar object. It is a third term, which is really two. It could be three, but it is the subject himself that occupies the third term.

AG   I agree, totally. I have described in one of the untranslated works something which I call the 'generalised triangular structure with variable third'. In other words, the structure is triangular but it doesn't mean that it is Oedipal. The third can be, for instance, art. It can be the body for a hypochondriac. But the important thing is to keep in mind that the third is always there, even though it is replaceable.

GK   Where the third term disappears, we have psychosis.

AG   Yes, indeed, in 'blank psychosis' I described a triangular situation in which, in fact, instead of having a father and a mother, we have two objects: the omnipotent malevolent one, and the weak benevolent one. So, it is one split in two, not only in terms of good and bad, but it is essential to see that while the bad is always certain, the good is always non-dependable. The bad one is always there, never loses, is never un-available, is never weak. The British told me a saying that we don't have in French: 'better the devil you know than the one you don't know', and *that* is better than no evil at all! There is a special attachment to the bad object, even though it's a malignant presence ... In the French tradition, since the contributions of Lacan, we always keep in mind the instance of the dead father, which means that the father is not only the person who is there, he is also the ancestors, the lost people of earlier generations which came to form the family, and so on. But I wonder, how about the mother? Why isn't there a dead mother like there is a dead father? The problem with the mother is entirely different. If we wanted to postulate the dead mother in a similar way, it wouldn't be the same; it wouldn't be the succession of mothers − the mother plus the mother of the mother, etc. The experience had to do with the lost object as irreplaceable, with no other substitute to it.

GK   You write in 'The dead mother' that there is an anxiety, but this is not about castration, i.e., it is not linked to the Oedipal; it's an anxiety about the lost object.

AG   The loss of the breast, which is in everybody, is a universal phenome-non. Now, in some instances, the loss becomes more dramatic. Why? I described the sudden depression of the mother, and here I make a differ-ence between the chronically depressed mother who is depressed from the beginning, and the normal situation with a mother who one day gets depressed. Two things interested me: one, nobody knows *why* the mother is depressed. The baby doesn't know it, and it is not sure that the others know it; in fact, there can be many reasons for the depression: perhaps a miscarriage, for instance (which is very, very frequent ... pro-voked or spontaneous). It can be the awareness of the mother that the father is cheating on her. It can be that she has lost her own father or mother. There are many possibilities; what is different here is that this depressed, dead mother doesn't disappear. She is still there and she is depressed, and that makes a tremendous change in the baby who doesn't understand what goes on. He loses the meaning of the relationship. The usual clinical descriptions of depression seem unaware of this, because they have always an explanation in terms of internal objects and so on, but most of the time what is conflictual and paradoxical in this situation is that everything continues to go on, and yet everything has changed.

GK   You make a distinction in this respect, between the loss of an object that produces depression, and the loss of an object which produces emptiness, the blank psychosis.

AG   Yes. All the states of emptiness have been discovered very late, fifty years ago or so; before, nobody spoke of them, you cannot find one sentence in Freud about it. The blank depression, the emptiness, all these states are related to states of decathexis. Cathexis and decathexis are great concepts and very useful ideas. If we don't use them, we do not understand anything. Cathexis is what makes your life continuous, good or bad, but still meaningful. When you undergo depression, you understand that what you thought were normal processes in life are loaded with cathexis. To wake up in the morning, to wash, to take one's breakfast, to go to work, or to read, all this means that you have a permanent flow of energy that you put in all these activities, of which you are unconscious, and which suddenly is not there any longer. You may become conscious of it if you are happy in some peculiar circumstances. As Winnicott says, the general mood is depressive except on holidays; you really discover cathexes when you have lost them. Because really, everything requires a tremendous effort. So this concept of energy (a concept which, actually, everyone rejects) is absolutely indispensable.

GK   You described two different movements in one same process: one movement is constituted by the disinvestment of the primary maternal object; and, at the same time, there is another movement, which is constituted by an identification with that object, the object is incorporated ...

AG   Without the subject knowing it. It is a paradox.

GK   Well, one can argue that the subject keeps the object somehow alive in himself or herself, although the object is dead; it constitutes a 'live' attachment to the deadness of the object. I don't know what you'll make of this, but here it is: in the same way that the dead father is a trans-generational phenomenon because the identification of the subject is with the parents' superego, (i.e. it is not with the actual parent), and this creates the possibility of the transmission of culture from one generation to the next, across three generational stages, there is also something trans-generational in the dead mother concept: most of the conflicts which make the mother 'dead' (while still alive) might be related to her conflicts with the previous generation: her mother, father, etc.

AG   I wouldn't say that, I would state it differently. We discussed the emphasis of the French on absence and the emphasis of the British on presence. The dead mother is one situation in which it is not so much the absence which comes into play, but really the presence with an absent mother.

GK   The dead presence.

AG   Yes. Now, you're right, the baby doesn't know that what worries the mother is, for instance, her relationship with her own mother. But even if this is true, it is the materialisation of this conflict in the relationship with the baby which is harmful. We see the difference. It is not something that the child is able to discover, it is not even a 'secret' in the family, it is really the direct relationship between mother and child which is here, somehow, wrong. Things are not how they should be. That's the difference. It is not an absence, like in the case of the dead father; it is a presence, even though it is a dead presence. I believe very much in this distinction made by Freud: on the one hand, the relationship to the present, which implies a contact, from body to body, the maternal body, the prototype of all future loving relationships; and, on the other hand, the relationship to the father as an identification which always involves the distance to the object – the fascination of the object, what it looks like, how it appears, but no direct contact. And I think that these are two dimensions of psychic development, which always have to be considered at the same time. We always have to consider what is the result of the relationship in terms of contact, bodily contact, and on the other hand, what we phantasise about a person who is there. The father doesn't need, in order to be present, to manifest himself in exceptional circumstances. The reasons for which he becomes a lovable object are surely different from what goes on with the other. As close as he may be with his children, he has no possibility of meeting the demands that are addressed to the mother. It might be exciting being with him, but it will never be the same kind of excitement – never mind the sex of the individual, whether it's a girl or a boy. This is the basis of a whole series of processes, starting from identification to the idealisation of the object.

GK   We seem to know so little about identification …

AG   There are so many different aspects of the process of identification; it is impossible to reduce it to just one concept, or one view of identification. For instance, it is of no use to understand identification as the Kleinians do, who speak of identification and object relationship as if they were interchangeable. Where is the specificity of identification in their view? You cannot find it. Freud gives a very progressive process of identification: in the beginning identification and the object relationship can replace one and the other, but in the end identification and the object relationship go opposite ways. If you have one, you cannot have the other. Desire means that the desire will be fulfilled when you will be able to reach the contact with the object. Identification is the tool. You won't have the object, but you will identify with the one who has it, which is, of course, a totally different process involving a detour. While the British school takes projective identification so much into account, the French extend the field of historic identification. Please, don't respond to me by saying that the first one is earlier.

GK   In terms of the dead mother again, there seems to be a paradox between the incapacity to find enjoyment that these subjects suffer from, and the enjoyment that creative people have in their creativity – even though they might have the dead mother syndrome.

AG   I had a poet in psychotherapy. He could not have an analysis – he was too ill for that. He stayed with me for six years; during three of those years, he couldn't write a word. And what can you do about *that* when you are an analyst? You can interpret, but it has no effect. When the writing starts again, nobody knows why; it comes at the most unexpected moment; it is not controllable. This is really the problem with creativity, among the people we see. Of course, you can bring back castration anxiety, but castration anxiety seems such a poor concept where you want to account for the inhibitions of creativity. What happens is really like the drying of a vital source. My patient used to tell me, '*Ça ne chante pas* – it didn't sing any more'. This is one of the most mysterious things: why the playing stops, or the song stops, or the vitality disappears. These subjects have chosen creativity over the love relationship, maybe to become independent from the object; the object, after all, can stop loving you; one moment, the object is there, at another moment, it has disappeared. There is a joy in creativity, but I think that there is this constant threat that you won't be able to go beyond.

GK   In creativity, there is no sharing. The sharing with others takes place at the level of narcissistic gratification, which is not the motivation for creating. I had a number of patients who were painters; a couple of them, who were quite accomplished, were also sexual perverts. For all of them, though, their creativity was much more important than their perversion ...

AG   It always is.

GK   ... and I don't think that this could be reduced to simply explaining it in terms of social acceptance. For some, it was touch and go; it could have gone one way or the other, perversion or creativity. But, whether artist or pervert, they both sometimes seem to share a refusal to mourn. I am not making a judgement about this, but there is a refusal of reality for the artist and for the pervert. Of course, in the case of the artist, thank God for that!

AG   The pervert and the artist refuse the world as it is. They both say, 'This is not the real world; the real world is what I am going to create.' But for the artist, he has to rely on what others before him have already created. There is no artist who is an absolute beginner – he always relates to some artist before him, some period, some school, even if it is with ambivalence, or to oppose it. There is recognition. The pervert wants to invent it all, right from the beginning. Maybe we too are like artists. We can't be absolute beginners, we have developed our own thinking through those that we admire, and also through those which we disagree with.

The important thing is our quest for trying to match experience and understanding.

GK Well, talking of beginnings ... we have come to the end of these interviews. Thank you very much.

AG Thank you.

Notes

1 *Un Psychanalyst Engagé – Conversation avec Manuel Macías*, Paris: Calman-Levy, 1994.
2 *André Green*, by François Dupare, Paris: Presses Universitaires de France, 1996.
3 *Jacques Lacan*, by Gilbert Diatkine, Paris: Presses Universitaires de France, 1997.
4 *Boundary and Space: An Introduction to the Work of D. W. Winnicott*, by Madeleine Davis and David Wallbridge, London: H. Karnac (Books) Ltd, 1981.
5 'Comments on the significance of Piaget's work for psychoanalysis', by A.-M. Sandler, *The International Journal of Psycho-Analysis*, 1975, 2: 4, 365–78.
6 *Bright Air, Brilliant Fire: On the Matter of the Mind*, by G. Edelman, New York: Basic Books, 1992.

2

PSYCHIC REALITY, NEGATION, AND THE ANALYTIC SETTING

Michael Parsons

'Maintaining an analytic stance' means actively holding on to a particular frame of mind. Most commonly it refers to how psychoanalysts are with their patients, but it also applies to the state of mind needed for thinking analytically or reading analytic writings. Whatever the situation, there is work involved in sustaining it. There is a sense of tension – slight, maybe, but constant. There is always a tug in the opposite direction, a pull away from the analytic state of mind. When we look at something which is not quite within our normal range of vision and try to focus on it, the muscles of accommodation in our eyes have to work harder than usual and we become conscious of keeping a steady tension in them as we work to keep the object in focus. It is not painful or difficult. We might not even call it a strain. But the effort, the tension, of not letting the focus slip, is there. Keeping oneself attuned to the realm of psychic reality rather than ordinary reality requires a particular sort of effort. There is a resistance to be overcome.

A patient told me about how, as a girl, she would be frightened of burglars in the night and wake her father up. He would reassure her that there weren't any burglars. This would make her more agitated, not less, and she would tell him she was afraid of dying, or of nuclear war. He would again reassure her, rather irritably now, that she was perfectly well, and there wasn't going to be a nuclear war. The reason this was so unhelpful to her is that she wanted him to meet her at the level of psychic reality where her fear was real, and the necessary question was, 'so what is she *really*, that is to say *psychically*, afraid of?' He, however, was meeting her in terms of ordinary reality which showed him, and made him say to her, that there was nothing really to be afraid of. In order to see that there *was* something to be afraid of, and then to think about what it might be, he would have had to negate his ordinary way of thinking.

Contrast this with Freud's attitude to the delusional self-reproaches of the melancholic. He says in 'Mourning and melancholia':

> It would be equally fruitless from a scientific and a therapeutic point of view to contradict a patient who brings these accusations against his ego. He must surely be right in some way and be describing something that is as it seems to him to be.
>
> (Freud, 1917, p. 246)

Freud is doing exactly what my patient's father could not do. He sets aside the automatic, ordinary response, 'That's absurd. Of course you're not like that!', and asks in what way it is not absurd. But this respect for reality at the psychic level is such an unusual, non-habitual way of thinking that it requires a distinct negating of our automatic attitudes.

It might be assumed that negating ordinary reality must be an avoidance, like denial or disavowal. Negation needs to be disentangled from those concepts. In his paper on negation Freud (1925) says clearly that negation is on the one hand defensive but also, on the other hand, important in freeing thinking from repression. The first part of this is familiar, but the second part tends to get forgotten. If negation is aligned with other concepts so as to make it automatically something counter-productive, this leaves no room for what Freud was pointing to.

This chapter considers how negation can sometimes be a way of avoiding reality, but also how the setting aside of ordinary reality is an essential element in all psychic work, particularly psychoanalytic work. What matters is how the underlying activity of negating is being used, whether to contradict reality or to disengage from it for the time being, without denying it.

Freud first mentions what he came to call psychic reality in the *Project*, where he writes: 'Indications of discharge through speech are also in a certain sense indications of reality – but of thought-reality not of external reality' (Freud, 1895, p. 373). In *The Interpretation of Dreams* he says: 'If we look at the unconscious wishes reduced to their most fundamental and truest shape we shall have to conclude, no doubt, that *psychical* reality is a particular form of existence not to be confused with *material* reality' (Freud, 1900, p. 620). In the *Introductory Lectures* he speaks of phantasies possessing '*psychical* as contrasted with *material* reality' (Freud, 1916–17, p. 368); and in the paper 'The Unconscious' he lists, as one of the characteristics of the system *Ucs.*, 'replacement of external by psychical reality' (Freud, 1915b, p.187). The striking thing is that in all these quotations psychic reality is defined by the negation of external, or material, reality. The father of the woman who was afraid of burglars would have needed, in order to understand her fears, to negate his own focus on ordinary reality in favour of her psychic reality. If staying in touch with psychic reality means sustaining the tension of negating ordinary reality, these texts suggest that this is not just an incidental necessity, but that it comes from an intrinsic connection between psychic reality and negation.

The first reaction to the idea of negating ordinary reality might be to see it as something defensive. Certainly, psychic reality may be used defensively. If ordinary reality is too painful or conflictual there can be a retreat from it into a psychic reality where those conflicts are, in one way or another, negated. The passage quoted above from the *Introductory Lectures* runs, in full: 'The phantasies possess *psychical* as contrasted with *material* reality, and we gradually learn to understand that *in the world of the neuroses it is psychical reality which is the decisive kind*' (Freud, 1916–17, p. 368). This clearly links psychic reality to pathology; the cure of the neurosis will lie in undoing the defensive negation of ordinary reality. In similar vein Freud describes how there may be 'a domination by an internal psychical reality over the reality of the external world and the path to a psychosis lies open' (Freud, 1939, p. 76).

Psychic reality, however, is not only a refuge from ordinary reality. The opposite may also be true. The starting-point for this chapter was how maintaining an analytic stance requires a resistance to the pull of ordinary reality so as to stay in the realm of psychic reality. Particularly when patients do *not* speak from their psychic reality but use *ordinary* reality defensively, the analyst must work all the harder to hold a position within psychic reality, knowing that that is where analytic work is done.

What Freud could do, and my patient's father could not, was to see what was being spoken about in terms of external reality – burglars, nuclear war, having committed some terrible crime – as being a representation of something that belonged to internal reality. This idea is fundamental, of course, to the whole of clinical psychoanalysis. A patient told me, for example, how the local businessmen in a particular community were getting together to improve the environment and develop the amenities in the area, and how different this was from somewhere else where the local people seemed unable to mobilise themselves and co-operate in that way. I took this as a description of his own internal state, and of his concern whether the different aspects of himself could come together so as to mobilise his own resources and bring about change in him. This is a commonplace enough interpretation, but it illustrates rather clearly the idea of external reality as a representation of internal reality.

What makes the interpretation possible is the analyst's being able to see external reality in this way, and to hold on to this understanding as a piece of psychic reality, against the pull of the ordinary meaning of the material. That is not to say that this patient was particularly resistant; he was not. But making any such interpretation means actively setting aside the first meaning of the material that presents itself. The patient must be able to do the same thing, if he is to understand and make use of the interpretation. So this constructive use of psychic reality involves the negating of ordinary reality, just as much as its defensive use does.

The passages from Freud, quoted above, were written years apart and do not hang together systematically. It is not clear whether Freud distinguishes between psychic and internal reality, nor whether ordinary, external and material reality are interchangeable concepts or have different connotations. The idea of psychic reality has been understood in such a variety of ways that it has become an ambiguous and somewhat problematical concept. A whole Congress of the International Psychoanalytical Association was devoted to elucidating it (IPA Congress, 1996); one contributor denied that the concept served any useful function at all (Arlow, 1996). The concept of psychic reality stays alive none the less, with observational studies of infant development focusing fresh attention on it (Fonagy and Target, 1996a, b; Emde *et al.*, 1997). My own emphasis here is to make a clear distinction between internal and psychic reality. Furthermore, the distinction between psychic and ordinary reality is not the same as the distinction between external and internal reality. Ordinary reality does refer to the encounters and events we experience in external reality. But the feelings, hopes and anxieties which comprise our internal experience are also part of our ordinary reality. These too are experiences we have, or which happen to us. By ordinary reality I mean the ensemble of our internal and external realities, as we experience them. Psychic reality is the realm where we *reflect* on what happens to us. Our psychic reality is constituted by what we *make* (consciously and unconsciously) of our experiences, both internal and external.

For that to happen, for us to have a psychic reality at all, some kind of representation of our experience is necessary. If we have no way of representing to ourselves what we experience, we cannot process it, and we are left with what Bion referred to as beta-elements and Lacan called the Order of the Real. Bion (1962, p. 3) resisted the idea of saying what alpha-function means, but I think it is very close to the capacity to represent our experience to ourselves, and thus to establish a psychic reality or, in Lacanian terms, the Symbolic Order. Psychic reality is the area where psychic work can be done, and not being able to establish it, for lack of alpha-function, is the mark of psychotic functioning and characterises those personalities described by Bion (1970, p. 9) who can only feel pain but not suffer it, and so cannot 'suffer' pleasure either. Psychic reality is constituted by finding ways of representing our experience to ourselves, and a large part of the work of psychoanalysis lies in helping the patient create a psychic reality out of ordinary reality, by discovering how to represent his experience to himself so that the psychical transformation of that experience becomes possible.

The point of a representation is that it is not the thing itself. It denotes what it is a representation of, but what allows experience to be processed is the separation between the representation in psychic reality and the thing itself in literal reality. The representation, in fact, is *instead of* the literal reality. Making use of the representation means setting aside, for the time being, the thing of which it is a representation, just as understanding the psychic reality of a patient's communication means setting aside the ordinary reality of its surface meaning.

There is a close connection, in this respect, between psychic reality and symbolism. As Freud's references to psychic reality stress the defensive aspect of it, so symbolism was seen to begin with as a form of regression (Jones, 1916, pp. 89–90; pp. 95–6 quoting Rank and Sachs), and was defined in terms of its defensive function. Jones wrote: 'That symbolism arises as the result of intrapsychical conflict between the repressing tendencies and the repressed is the view accepted by all psycho-analysts' (Jones, 1916, p. 115).

But psychic reality, with its negation of ordinary reality, also establishes a space in which psychic work can be done, and it was correspondingly recognised in due course that symbolism also has positive functions. Klein, for example, still seeing symbolism in terms of anxiety and conflict, nevertheless wrote: 'Thus, not only does symbolism come to be the foundation of all phantasy and sublimation but, more than that, it is the basis of the subject's relation to the outside world and to reality in general' (Klein, 1930, p. 221).

In a classic paper on symbol formation Milner described how

> [she had] … grown rather tired of being treated by this boy as his gas, his breath, his faeces … But when I began to see and to interpret, as far as I could, that this use of me might be not only a defensive regression, but an essential recurrent phase in the development of a creative relation to the world, then the whole character of the analysis changed; the boy then gradually became able to allow the external object, represented by me, to exist in its own right.
>
> (Milner, 1952, p. 104)

The importance of symbolism in developing a creative relationship to the world has since become generally accepted (Segal, 1957; Winnicott, 1967). This is not just a simple parallel between symbolism and psychic reality. A symbol is a particular kind of representation, and it has its symbolic function only in so far as it belongs to psychic reality. If the symbol does not exist in psychic reality, it is equated to the object in ordinary reality, in which case it cannot symbolise the object. There can only be, in Segal's (1957, p. 53) terms, a symbolic equation. The distinction between symbolisation and symbolic equation underlines the fact that although a symbol refers to the original object, its symbolic function depends on its being detached from it. The symbol at one and the same time points to the object and negates it as it exists in ordinary reality. Without that negation there is no symbolisation.

There is an issue which I shall mention in passing, in order to keep clear of it. A particular emphasis was given to the concept of representation, from the 1960s onwards, by Sandler and his co-workers at the Anna Freud Centre (Sandler, 1987, Chapters 4, 5, 15). Sandler's concept of the representational world has been much discussed. Whether it successfully clarifies such notions as internalisation, introjection, projection, and identification, whether or not representations have a motivating function, what connection they have with the drives: these and other questions have been argued over, particularly by ego-psychologists who see the idea of representation as a Trojan horse from the object-relations camp (Perlow, 1995, pp. 85–98). My present point, which is simply that reflecting on experience implies being able to represent it, is not part of that controversy.

The material from my patient about the local businessmen illustrated how external reality can represent internal reality. There is one external situation in psychoanalysis which functions in a very particular way as a representation of internal psychic structure, and that is the psychoanalytic situation itself. For the patient to come every day and lie on the couch free-associating, with the evenly attentive analyst seated behind, all within the framework of the session, is not only a way of finding access to the mind and its contents. It is that, of course, but one might call this the weak version of the point at issue. The strong version is that the structure of the analytic setting is itself a representation of internal mental structure. It not only gives access to internal structure; it embodies it.

If psychic reality is constituted by representation, and representation depends on an act of negation, that makes negation an essential element in the constitution of psychic reality. I want to suggest that an important feature of internal psychic functioning which is embodied in the structure of the psychoanalytic setting is the activity of negation. First, though, it may be helpful to illustrate, with the examples of the dream-state and the Oedipus complex, what it means to say that the external structure of the analytic setting represents aspects of an internal structure.

The analytic setting as a representation of the mind in a dream-state has been explored by several writers, notably Lewin (1955). He comments that the analytic setting arose historically out of the setting for hypnosis, Freud being led to develop it because certain patients proved not susceptible to the hypnotic state. So there was from the beginning a relation between the structure of the analytic setting and sleep, censorship and resistance. Despite the shift away from hypnosis, the analytic patient's narcissistic withdrawal of attention from the outside world still corresponds, says Lewin, to the narcissism of sleep, with its complete withdrawal of cathexis from external reality.

Lewin is using 'narcissism' not as a symptomatic description of pathology, but a metapsychological description of a self-absorbed state of mind. He observes that psychoanalytic interest in dreaming has centred on comparing the formation of dreams with the formation of neurotic symptoms, and on how mechanisms such as condensation and displacement are put to the same use in both. He points out that this comparison, which has been clinically so fruitful, has steered psychoanalysis away from its initial interest in the metapsychology of dreaming:

The study of the patient as a quasi-sleeper or quasi-dreamer was completely subordinated to the therapeutic and theoretical study of his symptoms ... The patient on the couch was *prima facie* a neurotic person and only incidentally a dreamer.

(Lewin, 1955, p. 169)

Freud himself commented that free association resembles the state of mind that precedes sleep (Freud, 1900, p. 102), and if the patient on the couch is a quasi-sleeper or a quasi-dreamer, it is free association that represents the uncensored activity of the unconscious, pushing forward to express material which in turn provokes censorship. The conflict between free association and resistance, so fundamental to the analytic setting, exactly represents the intra-psychic conflict and censorship that give rise to the latent and manifest content of dreams. One might also compare the analytic constraint against action to the neuromuscular inhibition during sleep, which makes possible the continuance of the dreaming state. The analyst, whose awareness makes bridges between the latent and the manifest material, is in the position of the sleeper's ego that can articulate the dream work, releasing and organising the unconscious wishes (Khan, 1974, p. 36). The analyst works in the reverse direction, however, trying to see through the defences, not keep them in place, and is therefore an 'awakener' rather than a guardian of sleep (Lewin, 1955).

André Green has also touched on the analytic setting and the dream-state but, in addition, has shown how the setting is a representation of the Oedipus Complex:

The symbolism of the setting comprises a triangular paradigm, uniting the three polarities of the *dream* (narcissism), of *maternal caring* (from the mother, following Winnicott) and of the *prohibition of incest* (from the father, following Freud). What the psychoanalytic apparatus gives rise to, therefore, is *the symbolisation of the unconscious structure of the Oedipus Complex*.

(Green, 1984, p. 123; translated for this edition by M. Parsons)

The first polarity is the dream situation. With the second and third of his polarities, Green points to another way in which the psychoanalytic framework is a representation of psychic structure. There are two different kinds of object that the analyst, by virtue of the setting, represents. One aspect of the analytic situation is the peaceful, reliable environment, the lying down, the invitation to say anything and express any wish or feeling, without censoring it. The analyst who offers these is inviting the patient to regress and be cared for in a state of dependence. But there are other aspects, such as the prohibition on enacting wishes or feelings, the rigour and constraints about session times and payment of fees, and the analyst's refusal to accept at face value what the patient offers him. This is what Friedman (1997, p. 30) calls the 'adversarial' quality of analysis, and the analyst who embodies it is a different object for the patient from the one that offers regression. The analyst thus represents two opposite sorts of object at the same time. The patient's wish is to separate them out and to be able to relate to one of them but not the other. But these two objects have their own relationship with each other. There is a union between them in the person of the analyst, which the patient is not privy to. The patient has to accept this, and find a way of relating to both of them together, despite the wish to keep them apart and establish a special relationship with just one.

These two objects are both located, in their externalised forms, in the analyst, but they are also fundamental to the structure of the patient's internal world. The nature of the analytic framework sets up a triangle of conflict between them and the patient, and thus represents in its own structure the unconscious structure of the Oedipus complex, just as it does the internal state of the dreamer.

These examples of the dreaming state and the Oedipus complex show what it means for the structure of the psychoanalytic situation to be an external representation of internal psychic structure. Here is some clinical material to indicate that, in the same way, the analytic setting is an external representation of the negating which is essential to the creation of psychic reality.

A woman started four times weekly analysis, not responding to my invitation to use the couch but sitting opposite me in the chair. The reason she gave for seeking help was uncertainty about whether to have a baby. Her way of talking was bright, cheerful, often laughing; but her cheerfulness felt brittle and defensive and an underlying unhappiness was evident. She prattled on, with few pauses and no real silences, and was noticeably unreflective about herself. I was not at all clear what she wanted from me, and when I made an interpretative, or at least a linking, kind of comment, she would consider it briefly, say something like 'Yes, well …', and rush back into a narrative of her busy day or complaints about her husband. For several weeks I was struck by how thoroughly she seemed to avoid thinking about what she was doing in coming to see me. When I brought up the idea of the couch again she dismissed it, mentioning in passing that the couch looked like a bed. Shortly afterwards, in a different context, she made a reference to platonic relationships. It seemed the couch aroused too strong a sexual anxiety of some, as yet unknown, nature.

She became pregnant and was uncertain whether she wanted to keep the baby. She did not want to discuss it with her GP, for fear he would take her into some back room of his surgery and want to do an abortion himself on the spot. She knew this was unrealistic, but when eventually she saw an obstetrician there was a similar fear about letting him examine her. She did not know what he might suddenly want to do next. There did not seem to be any clear or specific fantasy, but her anxiety was powerful. By this time I had been able to make some references to the relationship between us, so when this material about the GP and the obstetrician appeared I said that I now understood that her reaction to the couch showed the same anxiety about what I might secretly have in mind to do with her. She came in to the next session and, without saying anything, immediately lay down on the couch.

I was startled, not just by her doing this, but by the instantly noticeable change in how she talked and, even more, in the whole quality of her presence. On her second day on the couch her session went as follows. She said that she suddenly felt like going to sleep; then, ironically, that it would be an expensive sleep! I said that all the same she was probably talking about something she did feel she needed. She said that at home she certainly would not be able to lie down and have an hour to herself. (Pause.) She said she had stretched some of the canvases she had bought (she is an artist). Should she stick to her plan of getting them all stretched first, or start a painting now on one of the stretched ones? (Pause.) She said that sometimes, out driving, she just takes a turning on impulse, even if it is not where she is meant to be going. I said something about finding her own direction as she went along. There was a considerable silence. She said, rather suddenly, that this was very different from sitting up. I made a questioning sound, and she said 'Less like conversation'. When she used to sleep over with one of her school friends, they would lie in their beds in the dark, just talking about anything, until his mother came in and told them to shut up. All this was in a slow and reflective, almost meditative, vein. I noted that the school friend, like myself, was male. The bedroom, a potentially sexual place that seemed safe for the time being, might represent the analytic room. There was also the anxiety about someone who might try and put a stop to this new way of talking and being. There seemed no need at this point, though, to interrupt her new-found free associating with interpretations.

She recalled talking yesterday about whether to go on seeing the same obstetrician. It was as much to do with the traffic and parking problems around his workplace, as about whether she thought he was a good doctor or not. Well, she said, she had decided like that about coming to see me too. She had always liked my road, for the way it sits rather hidden between two others. She liked the room, the feel of its space. Spaces were important to her. Another analyst she had consulted had a sink in the consulting room; she didn't like that. Doctors always had sinks, full of instruments and junk. I said here was the same concern again, about what the doctor might do. What would the junk in the sink be for? She said she had seen things pretty clearly in the other analyst's sink, but she was sure there wasn't anything there really.

There was a photo in yesterday's paper of a murder victim, looking beautiful and innocent, with a story that she had in fact been a violent and cruel character. It reminded her of a Cindy Sherman work (an artist whose works contain disturbing images of the artist herself). She said she can never draw herself except in the mirror. I said that she might be afraid of what would appear as she drew herself, unless she looked in the mirror for reassurance. She went back to the school friend, whom she still sees. He could always give things a humorous turn. Even a serious conversation with him, about her pregnancy, had had laughs in it. Maybe she would phone him. But he usually had his answering machine on. What if he didn't pick up, and just left her talking? As she said this she turned on her front, on the couch, and looked at me. I said I thought I had picked up her message. Lying on the couch not seeing me, she was worried whether I was really there for her, listening and willing to respond. I thought as well that she was looking to see in what way I would respond and what instruments I might be planning to use. For serious talk with me to be safe, that would matter a lot.

Beyond the particular interpretation I also had a sense that she was asking if I could pick up that *kind* of message, if I was ready for this allusive, associative way of communicating. After the preceding weeks, this abrupt change in tonality as she moved from the chair to the couch was as distinct as a suddenly different taste in the mouth. Unmistakably, this was the experience of shifting from ordinary reality into psychic reality. There is, of course, a reciprocity in this. She finds a way of doing what the father of my first patient could not do, and she wonders whether I am ready for this shift. But when she makes her move from ordinary to psychic reality, it not only means that she can talk differently; it also helps my own efforts to occupy psychic reality, so that I am able to listen differently.

When she lay on the couch for the first time, the way she did it, immediately on entering the room and without explanation, felt like an active negation of what had been going on before. There was another key moment, when she was struck by how different lying on the couch felt from sitting up. It was 'less like conversation'. Again, this is a recognition of the negative. With the disappearance of something which belongs to ordinary, sitting-up, conversation-like reality, space is made for something different. This is simple and apparently obvious, but I want to highlight its significance. Specific aspects of the analytic situation are regularly understood in terms of their function. Lying down, for example, helps towards a regressive state of mind. Coming four or five times a week encourages an intensity of transference experience, and makes it harder for defences to be constantly re-established. The profound silence of the analyst brings anxieties into the open. Such observations are true enough but, more generally, the lying down, the frequency and the silence are all examples of how the analytic situation is set up so as to embody the negation of ordinary reality.

This has corollaries when it comes to variations on the setting. There is a familiar debate about whether fewer than four or five sessions a week is a satisfactory analytic situation. Among the many subtle arguments that have been brought forward, it is worth saying that to have more frequent sessions is, quite simply, *more different* from ordinary conversational reality. Lying down to talk to someone you cannot see might be a still greater negation of ordinary reality than talking face to face, however frequent that was. If someone is coming less often, maybe only twice or once a week, it tends to be seen as less appropriate to use the couch. But if the sessions are less frequent, it might be *more* important to use the couch, provided the patient can tolerate it, because that is how ordinary reality can still be emphatically negated. This would keep the therapeutic situation still representing as much as possible the negation of ordinary reality.

There is an interesting episode in the history of psychoanalysis in Japan. This was pioneered by Heisaku Kosawa who studied with Freud in Vienna in the 1930s, being analysed by Richard Sterba and supervised by Paul Federn. Back in Japan he began analysing patients in the conventional way using the couch. Later he stopped using it regularly and often saw patients sitting up; but not face to face. He still sat out of sight, with the patient's chair turned away from him. Analyst and patient sat in their chairs, both facing in the same direction with the analyst behind. Strange as this may seem, and whatever Kosawa's reasons for giving up the couch, the clinical situation he did use still shows, to my mind, a fine awareness of the need to negate ordinary reality. If the analytic setting represents in its external structure the internal activity of negation, and if, as I argued earlier, negation is essential to the creation of psychic reality, this means that the structure of the analytic situation represents the process by which psychic reality is constituted. We are looking, in fact, at what makes the psychoanalytic situation psychoanalytic.

The comparison of psychic reality and symbolism showed the same double function in both of them. Both can be used defensively to avoid contact with ordinary reality, but they are also both essential to an alive engagement with it. The reason for this is that they both depend intrinsically on negation; and negation itself has a double function. It can be used in different, opposing, ways, and the use to which the act of negation is being put, is what determines whether psychic reality or symbolism is being used defensively or constructively.

Freud's (1925) paper on negation investigates exactly this question of its double function. Freud introduces negation as a clearly defensive procedure. 'Now you'll think I mean to say something insulting, but really I've no such intention.' 'You ask who this person in the dream can be. It's *not* my mother' (Freud, 1925, p. 235). A page later, however, Freud is writing: 'With the help of the symbol of negation, thinking frees itself from the restrictions of repression and enriches itself with material that is indispensable for its proper functioning' (ibid., p. 236). Negation frees thinking from repression, Freud says, because the people who say 'I'm not insulting you' or 'It's not my mother' are letting themselves be aware of something they might have completely obliterated – the aggression, the association with mother – by virtue of saying that it does not count for anything. In itself that is defensive, but it does at least allow the thing in question out of the unconscious and makes it available for thinking about. In that way negation is 'a way of taking cognizance of what is repressed' (ibid., p.235). The essential factor in this is that

> the intellectual function is separated from the affective process. With the help of negation only one consequence of the process of repression is undone – the fact, namely, of the ideational content of what is repressed not reaching consciousness. The outcome of this is a kind of intellectual acceptance of the repressed, while at the same time what is essential to the repression persists.
>
> (ibid., p. 236)

For Freud this thought was by no means new. It is a thread running through his work from *Jokes and their Relation to the Unconscious* (1905), through 'The two principles of mental functioning' (1911), and the metapsychological papers 'Repression' (1915a) and 'The unconscious' (1915b) up to this paper in 1925. In all those he refers to the connection between intellectual judgement and repression, with the idea gradually emerging that conflictual experience can be saved from repression and be available for thinking about, if the emotional aspect of the conflict is separated from its intellectual evaluation. Freud's concern was with intellectual judgement, but the converse must also be true of affective awareness. Clinical work in psychoanalysis shows all the time that for someone to stay in touch with feeling, and to let the nature of an emotional state reveal itself, it may be necessary to make the same separation between affective process and intellectual function. This way round, however, it is the intellectual awareness that has to be kept repressed in order for the emotion itself to become conscious. My patient's anxiety over doctors and their instruments, for example, could be conscious on condition that she did not know what it was about. This is the converse of what Freud described, but it depends on the same act of negation.

A tangential thought at this point. There is a tag to the effect that 'hysterics cannot think and obsessionals cannot feel'. Perhaps the underlying problem is that hysterics cannot negate their affect, so as to be able to think, and obsessionals cannot negate the ideational component so as to have access to their affect. Should we say, 'hysterics cannot stop feeling and obsessionals cannot stop thinking'?

After describing the negation which allows ideational content but not affect into consciousness, Freud says that one can sometimes succeed in 'conquering the negation as well, and in bringing about a full intellectual acceptance of the repressed' (Freud, 1925, p. 236). The double function of negation, however, shows that it is not so much a question of conquering negation as of how it is being used in the first place. If negation is being used to establish psychic reality as a realm for developing an engagement with the world, it will not need to be conquered. If, on the other hand, it is being used to establish psychic reality as a defensive structure, efforts to reduce it will indeed be treated as attempts at conquest and be resisted as such. The difference lies in whether negation is a fixed state to be held on to, or a mobile and flexible activity, a provisional suspension of ordinary reality to be moved on from when it has served its purpose. Negation may be used to contradict ordinary reality, or it may be used to disengage from it for the time being, without contradiction. The second of those makes it possible to work with the psychic representation instead of the real object, so as to come back to the real object in a new way. The former use of negation sets up a defensive psychic reality to be used as a refuge; the latter use sets up a psychic reality that extends the range of, and enriches, contact with ordinary reality.

The double usage of negation and the double function of psychic reality is related to what André Green has called 'the work of the negative'. This concept is developed in his book *Le Travail du négatif* (Green, 1993), and it sheds light on what it means for the use of negation to be free or restricted. All ego-development and any experiencing of ourselves as subjects has to be achieved against an essential background of loss and of absence. We become who we are by how we deal with the fact that we cannot have what we want nor be who we wish to be. Many psychoanalytic ideas need to be understood, according to Green, in terms of how they address this fundamental experience of lack. In considering the *fort–da* game at the beginning of *Beyond the Pleasure Principle* (Freud, 1920, pp. 14–16), for example, his emphasis would not be first on the *da*, the child's successful recovery of the cotton-reel, or his mother, but on the *fort*, his throwing away of the cotton-reel which is the acknowledgement that his mother is missing. The phrase 'the work of the negative' refers to how we cope with this inevitability of lacking what we want.

Depending on how we do cope with it, the work of the negative may take two different forms (Green, 1993, pp. 21, 244). One has a structuring effect on the ego and promotes development. The other is destructuring and hampers development. Demands to give something up are of many sorts: the infant's not being able to feed the instant it is hungry; failure to achieve an ambition; bereavement by the death of someone beloved. Bearing the loss or deprivation means facing the reality of the absence of the loved, or wished-for, object, or accepting the truth of not being like one's ideal. If it is possible to make the act of negation, to face the reality of lack, of absence, that opens the door, through a process of working-through, to new experience, new object-relationships and new ideals. This is the structuring form of the work of the negative. The same process, in microcosm, is continually at work in what I have been calling the constructive use of negation. All exploration of reality, all movement towards new experiences or new ways of being, all creativity and any kind of symbolic functioning, in fact the whole fabric of

71

psychic development, implies an ability to negate ordinary reality in favour of psychic reality.

Doing this depends on a trust in being able to work through to a new connection with ordinary reality. If there is too much unconscious anxiety about ever being able to do that, this way of using negation may not be possible. Then the truth of loss and absence cannot be faced, displacement and symbolisation are not possible, and negation can only be used to contradict the reality that cannot be borne. This different use of negation, by not being able to give up that which has been lost, or which cannot be had, fixes the negative and insists on it, in a way that keeps the door closed to any new experience or development. This is the opposite form of the work of the negative, which is destructuring and disorganising to the ego.

This destructuring use of negation is exemplified in Green's (1983) paper 'The dead mother'. He considers the situation of a mother who is absorbed by a bereavement, but who cannot give up that which is no longer there. The classic case involves the death of a child in infancy. The child's life and the mother's relationship with the living child have been negated by death. But the mother cannot allow that; she can only use the function of negation to contradict the truth of it. So she becomes frozen into a relationship with the negative of the child's existence. As Green (1993, p. 18) points out, this is, in Bion's (1970, p. 17) terms a relationship to a 'no-thing'. If nothing is there any more, accepting the negation of what was there is necessary for relationships to new things to become possible. Failing that, the nothing that is there may itself become the object. This is what happens with the dead mother, who makes a relationship to the 'no-thing' that is constituted by the absence of the dead child.

Green's term for this is 'negative hallucination'. He instances (Green, 1997) the patient described by Winnicott (1971, p. 23) who said to Winnicott about her previous analyst 'The negative of him is more real than the positive of you'. A woman who came to me for consultation presented another example. She was in psychotherapy at the time and experiencing great frustration in the therapeutic relationship. She understood about the idea of transference but felt the situation was so unproductive that she was considering breaking off treatment. A crucial episode in her life history had been a passionate love affair with an artist. He had ended the relationship and done so, as she felt, very brutally. When she said she had never got over it, she meant it in a very specific way. Although they had not seen each other for years and he was now married and living elsewhere, she said that in her mind the relationship was still just as much in existence today as ever. As we talked it became clear that she was indeed still actively involved in a relationship; but what she was relating to was the void this man had left behind, the gone-ness of what there had once been. He had created, when the relationship broke up, a work of art which, in its particular medium, powerfully embodied his rejection of her. The continued existence of this work of art helped perpetuate in her mind the active, continuing non-existence of the relationship. It was the embodiment of the negative of the relationship, and it was this negative that she was still relating to. The relationship to her therapist as a transference object could not compete with the active aliveness of her relationship to the negative of her ex-lover.

The constructive work of the negative requires a certain mobility, a capacity to shift between negating and affirming, separation and connection. Broadly speaking, the ability to use negation in this provisional, flexible way, so as to establish a creative kind of psychic reality, is an index of well-being. But of course there is nothing cut and dried about it. Everybody lies somewhere along a spectrum in their use of negation, and no doubt shifts up and down it from time to time. In his sequence of references to the relation between judgement and repression, Freud is trying to say something about an ebb and flow between different states of mind. We cannot be continuously in touch with the fullness of our experience at all levels, intellectual and emotional. We regularly need to distance ourselves from some part of our experience in order to address other parts, and to resolve conflicts. As a particular resolution is worked through it becomes possible to reconnect, we hope more richly, with what we had negated and enter again into the fullness of our experience; until the next time. The depth and quality of our emotional and thinking life thus move to a kind of tidal rhythm, which we may sense both in the short term, within a single hour or day, and over the years.

The analytic situation opens that rhythm, of movement and fixity in how patients negate and reconnect with their experience, to a unique kind of exploration. Furthermore, analysts too are now in touch, now out of touch with their own experience of the session. All analysts know what it is like to feel slow in the uptake. It is chastening to have the penny suddenly drop about what a patient has been trying to convey for a long time. I realised recently that one of my patients was telling me he felt an entire fun-loving, risk-taking side of his personality had been, to use his word, 'engineered' out of existence. Given the decades over which that had happened, and also his present life circumstances, he could see no possibility of ever recovering it. That part of him seemed gone for ever. When the impact of this hit me I thought 'How could I not have understood?!' But I think the sense of tragedy was such that I had to negate the affect (unconsciously at the time) in order first to grasp at an intellectual level what I was hearing about. Only later could I let the full emotional significance of it emerge, and begin to speak out of that awareness.

The psychoanalytic situation makes possible its unique exploration of unconscious mental life by virtue of the fact that its structure, in various different ways, is a representation in external reality of the internal structure it is investigating. This internal structure is thus both unconscious and made visible and audible at the same time. In particular, the analytic setting is an external representation of the internal negation which is essential to the establishing of psychic reality. The quality of a person's psychic reality, and the degree of freedom in his or her use of negation, will find a direct representation in the quality of the psychoanalytic situation that person can take part in, and in the degree of freedom with which he or she can use its negations of ordinary reality. The more restricted someone is to a fixed and immobilising use of negation, the more the analytic setting will represent, and draw the analyst into, a fixed and immobilised psychic reality; and the more difficult will be the analytic task of establishing a psychic reality in which the constructive work of the negative can take place.

A refinement, however, is needed to conclude with. It is incomplete to say that what makes the psychoanalytic situation psychoanalytic is its being a representation of psychic structure. That is true as far as it goes, but the analytic situation is not a static tableau. By its nature it calls on patients to express themselves, and on the patient and analyst to engage with each other. This makes the analytic situation not just a representation of psychic structure but an expression of it. It is the way psychic structure expresses itself, and cannot not express itself, through the structure of the setting, that makes the psychoanalytic situation psychoanalytic. This is what makes the unconscious visible and audible. The point is not that the analyst looks for something from the patient, within the setting. The analytic setting itself, by its very nature, constitutes a demand for the expression of the psychic apparatus; and this, as André Green (1984, p. 119) has put it, is what makes the setting a psychoanalytic apparatus.

References

Arlow, J. (1996) The concept of psychic reality – how useful? *International Journal of Psycho-analysis*, 77: 659–66.

Bion, W. (1962) *Learning from Experience*. London: Heinemann. Reprinted in *Seven Servants*. New York: Aronson, 1977.

—— (1970) *Attention and Interpretation: A Scientific Approach to Insight in Psycho-Analysis and Groups*. Reprinted in *Seven Servants*. New York: Aronson, 1977.

Emde, R., Kubicek, L. and Oppenheim, D. (1997) Imaginative reality observed during early language development. *International Journal of Psycho-analysis*, 78: 115–33.

Fonagy, P. and Target, M. (1996a) Playing with reality: I. Theory of mind and the normal development of psychic reality. *International Journal of Psycho-analysis*, 77: 217–33.

——(1996b) Playing with reality: II. The development of psychic reality from a theoretical perspective. *International Journal of Psycho-analysis*, 77: 459–79.

Freud, S. (1895) *Project for a Scientific Psychology. S. E.* 1: 295–397.

—— (1900) *The Interpretation of Dreams. S. E.* 4–5: xxiii–621.

—— (1905) *Jokes and Their Relation to the Unconscious. S. E.* 8: 9–238.

—— (1911) Formulations on the two principles of mental functioning. *S. E.* 12: 218–26.

—— (1915a) Repression. *S. E.* 14: 146–58.

—— (1915b) The unconscious. *S. E.* 14:166–204.

—— (1916–17) *Introductory Lectures on Psycho-Analysis. S. E.* 15–16: 9–463.

—— (1917) Mourning and melancholia. *S. E.* 14: 243–58.

—— (1920) *Beyond the Pleasure Principle. S. E.* 18: 7–64.

—— (1925) Negation. *S. E.* 19: 235–9.

——. (1939) *Moses and Monotheism: Three Essays. S. E.* 23: 7–137.

Friedman, L. (1997) Ferrum, ignis and medicina: return to the crucible. *Journal of the American Psychoanalytic Association*, 45: 21–36.

Green, A. (1983) The dead mother. In *On Private Madness*. London: the Hogarth Press, 1986, pp. 142–73.

—— (1984) Le langage dans la psychanalyse. In *Langages: Rencontres Psychanalytiques d'Aix-en-Provence 1983*. Paris: Les Belles Lettres, pp. 19–250.

—— (1993) *Le Travail du négatif*. Paris: Editions de Minuit.

—— (1997) The intuition of the negative in *Playing and Reality. International Journal of Psycho-analysis*, 78: 1071–84.

IPA Congress (1995) 39th Congress of the International Psychoanalytical Association, San Francisco, July–August 1995. Pre-published papers, *International Journal of Psycho-analysis*, 76: 1–49.

—— (1996) 39th Congress of the International Psychoanalytical Association, San Francisco, July–August 1995. Plenary papers and panel reports. *International Journal of Psycho-Analysis*, 77: 1–148.

Jones, E. (1916) The theory of symbolism. In *Papers in Psychoanalysis*, 5th edn. London: Baillière, 1948, pp. 87–144.

Khan, M. M. R. (1974) *The Privacy of the Self*. London: Hogarth Press.

Klein, M. (1930) The importance of symbol-formation in the development of the ego. In *The Writings of Melanie Klein*, vol. 1, London: Hogarth Press, 1975, pp. 219–32.

Lewin, B. (1955) Dream psychology and the analytic situation. *Psychoanalytic Quarterly*, 24: 169–99

Milner, M. (1952) The role of illusion in symbol formation. In *The Suppressed Madness of Sane Men: Forty-Four Years of Exploring Psychoanalysis*. London: Tavistock, 1987, pp. 83–113.

Perlow, M. (1995) *Understanding Mental Objects*. London: Routledge.

Sandler, J. (1987) *From Safety to Superego*. London: Karnac.

Segal, H. (1957) Notes on symbol formation. In *The Work of Hanna Segal*. New York: Aronson, 1981, pp. 49–65.

Winnicott, D.W. (1967) The location of cultural experience. In *Playing and Reality*. London: Tavistock, 1971, pp. 95–103.

—— (1971) *Playing and Reality*. London: Tavistock.

3

THE DEAD MOTHER SYNDROME AND THE RECONSTRUCTION OF TRAUMA

Arnold H. Modell

André Green's paper 'The dead mother' (Green, 1983) can be used as a paradigm of the child's response to a traumatic disruption of maternal relatedness in infancy and early childhood. This paper therefore raises certain fundamental epistemological questions regarding the reconstruction of the past, and the relation between trauma in infancy and early childhood and subsequent psychopathology. The dead mother syndrome can therefore be seen as a model that illuminates some elemental issues that are germane to both the practice and theory of psychoanalysis. It is a base from which we can explore the epistemology of trauma and the problem of reconstruction.

It may be useful to distinguish the dead mother *syndrome* from the dead mother *complex*. The term *dead mother syndrome* can be used to denote the intensely malignant clinical syndrome that Green described when there is a primary identification with the emotionally dead mother whereas the term *dead mother complex* denotes an entire range of an individual's response to a chronically depressed, emotionally absent mother. For example, Guntrip – in his well-known paper 'My experience of analysis with Fairbairn and Winnicott' – reports that he reconstructed with Winnicott his experience of a depressed and emotionally unrelated mother but he himself did not suffer from the dead mother syndrome (Guntrip, 1975). He suffered from a dead mother complex which in his case did not lead to emotional deadness (an identification with this mother) but to a hypersensitivity to schizoid states of withdrawal in others. To put the matter simply: everyone with a dead mother complex does not develop a dead mother syndrome. A mother's affective withdrawal from her infant and young child is a relatively common occurrence, whereas the dead mother syndrome, that bespeaks severe psychopathology, is quite rare. The variability of an individual's response to an emotionally absent mother illustrates the importance of a selective process within the individual as a response to trauma. I use the term *selection* in a Darwinian sense; it does not signify a conscious voluntary choice.

The phenomenology of the dead mother syndrome

In describing the internalization of the dead mother, André Green judiciously used the term *imago* to refer to the *patient's* construction or internal representation of the mother, which is not necessarily equivalent to the memory of the historical mother. The term imago denotes an unconscious identification. Nevertheless, the question of the historical mother cannot be totally evaded by the use of the term imago. The question of the historical mother still remains. The problem of an historical reconstruction of the mother's relatedness and affective state is complicated by the fact that as analysts we tend to identify with our patient's imagoes. And such sympathetic identification is probably a necessary ingredient of the therapeutic process. We form a corresponding image in our minds of the patient's mother to whom we may attribute the patient's psychopathology.

If we put aside those patients who are overtly psychotic, the dead mother syndrome remains one of the most difficult therapeutic problems that an analyst can encounter. I can confirm most of the salient features of the phenomenology of the dead mother syndrome that Green has portrayed. However, my own experience differs from that of Green's in one significant aspect. Green reports that in a successful analysis the patient may recover memories of a period of aliveness that preceded the mother's depression. My own cases suggest a somewhat different scenario: the mother's deadness is not experienced as a discrete episode with a beginning and an end, so that I have not been able to recover memories of a period where the mother was emotionally available. From the perspective of the *patient's* reconstruction of their mother, the mother may be perceived as someone with a permanent characterological deficit, rather than remembering their mother as having suffered from a time-limited depression. Furthermore, in some cases my patients do not necessarily recognise the mother's depression as such. In some cases, it is necessary that the analyst reconstruct that the mother was in fact depressed and emotionally absent. This has important therapeutic consequences, for otherwise patients may continue to believe that their mother turned away from them because of their intrinsic defectiveness or badness.

In some instances it would appear as if their mother was unable to recognise that her child had an inner life that was separate and distinct from her own. The mother was experienced as if she lacked the capacity to recognise other minds. The consequences of experiencing this failure of the mother to acknowledge the child's inner life can be devastating. For recognising the uniqueness of children's inner life is equivalent to recognising that they are psychically alive. It is as if their mothers failed to acknowledge their humanity. It is a short step to think that if their mother does not recognise their psychic aliveness, then their mother wishes that they did not exist, that they in fact should be dead.

If a child is not entitled to have an inner life that is unique and separate from that of the mother, it is as if the child has not been granted the permission to be a person. The failure to recognise the child's psychic aliveness may be felt by the child as the mother's withholding permission to exist. Believing that the mother withholds permission to exist may result in the conviction that all desires are forbidden, for if one does not have a right to exist, one has no right to have desires, to want anything for oneself.

Daniel Stern, in his paper 'One way to build a clinically relevant baby', acknowledges that he has been influenced by Green's concept of the dead mother when he described an analogous state in infancy. He observed the infant's 'micro-depression' resulting from its failed attempts to bring the mother back to life:

> Compared to the infant's expectations and wishes, the depressed mother's face is flat and expressionless. She breaks eye contact and does not seek to re-establish it. There is less contingent responsiveness. There is a disappearance of her animation, tonicity, and so on. Along with these invariants coming from the mother, there are resonant invariants invoked in the infant: the flight of animation, a deflation of posture, a fall in positive affect and facial expressivity, a decrease in activation, etc. In sum, the experience is descriptively one of a 'micro-depression'.
>
> (Stern, 1994, pp. 12–13)

The disruptive effects of the mother's unresponsiveness have also been demonstrated experimentally by Tronick (1989).

Stern goes on to say that 'After the infant's attempt to invite and solicit the mother to come to life, to be there emotionally, to play, have failed, the infant, it appears, tries to be with her by way of identification and imitation' (1994, p.13). This observation is consistent with Green's report that his patients suffered from a primary identification with the dead mother. It is as if the patient is saying: 'If I cannot be loved by my mother, I will become her'. I have found this total (primary) identification with the mother, in female patients, to be a salient feature of the dead mother syndrome that differentiates the dead mother syndrome from the dead mother complex. Many patients avoid the dead mother syndrome by a counter-identification, becoming the opposite of their mother, or believing that only a 'part' of themselves is dead, thus retaining a sense of individuality and preserving a self/object distinction. In contrast, in cases of primary identification the patient's individuality is completely lost as she becomes submerged within the mother that she has constructed. This construction of the mother's personality may consist of an internalisation, not of the mother's conscious attributes, but what the child experiences of mother's unstated and unconscious attitudes. For example, a mother who appears to the world to be a 'nice person' is perceived by her daughter to be filled with hatred, and accordingly the patient identifies with this presumed aspect of the mother and appears to be 'nice' but underneath feels hateful. This is a kind of ironic overcompensation: the mother ignores the daughter's inner life but the daughter, in turn, models herself on what she perceives as her mother's unconscious attitudes. This total identification with a dead mother who is incapable of loving, contributes to a corresponding incapacity to love others and to love oneself.

There is another aspect of the phenomenology of the dead mother syndrome that needs to be mentioned. This relates to the processing of affects. It is commonly recognized that a disturbance in the early mother/infant or mother/child relationship contributes to a relative incapacity to regulate affects. This is based on the recognition that in infancy homeostatic processes are mutually regulated (Beebe et al., 1997; Shore, 1994). This disturbance in affect regulation may arise from a non-specific asynchrony in the mother/child relationship, consistent with Bion's theory that the mother is the container and initial processor of the child's anxiety. One observes the fear of experiencing intense feelings with the belief that, inasmuch as affects are inherently uncontrollable, the self would be flooded and overwhelmed. If the mother is emotionally unresponsive, one may infer that she has distanced herself from her body and bodily experiences. If this should prove to be the case, this dissociation between the self and the body will be communicated to the child, and the mother will therefore prove to be relatively unable to facilitate the child's processing of his/her own affective experiences.

As I noted, this disturbance in affect processing is part of the dead mother syndrome, and I suspect an invariant accompaniment of that syndrome, but is also present in a wider range of disorders. What may be more specific to the dead mother syndrome is an inability to experience pleasure. This is different from what is ordinarily understood as a masochistic compulsion to seek pain. Pleasure itself, the pleasure of simply being alive, is missing. More than that, in some instances, pleasure that can be derived from any source, no matter how innocent, is forbidden. If pleasure is inadvertently experienced it must be punished.

Stern introduced a concept that I have found very useful in thinking about the problem of the dead mother. He speaks of a 'schema-of-being-with' (Stern, 1994). This is an inferential relational schema regarding the subjective state of an infant who is faced with being with a depressed mother. This term schema-of-being-with encompasses more that the static and one-dimensional term representation. The term schema-of-being-with intends to conceptualise the internalisation of a state of relatedness (or non-relatedness), a dynamic interaction. This schema can be used as paradigm for the chronic trauma that is the result of a disturbed mother/child relationship. The schema-of-being-with applies not only to developmental disturbances but can be a useful way of thinking of certain aspects of the transference in the adult patient. Those patients who suffer from the dead mother syndrome evidence great difficulties in 'being with the other'. Green alluded to this when he commented that 'the patient is strongly attached to the analysis more than the analyst' (Green, 1983, p.161). The patient does not know how to be with the analyst. In some cases it is felt to be dangerous to even acknowledge a relationship with the analyst, in spite of the fact, as Green observed, that they may be very devoted to the analysis itself. Any feeling of love for the analyst is felt to be dangerous and potentially destructive. Hence they become dead and lifeless in the analytic setting. They maintain a corpse-like posture, do not move on the couch, and speak in a dead-seeming voice drained of all affective valences. This deadness may prove to be contagious and infect the analyst who may find himself, or herself, also speaking in a dull lifeless monotone. The dead mother is a ghost which pervades the entire analytic process.

The problem of reconstruction

Questions regarding the truth or validity of psychoanalytic reconstructions and their etiological implications have been with us since the birth of psychoanalysis. The controversy is not static, as the intellectual and scientific environment that we all inhabit is constantly evolving. Those ambient scientific disciplines which influenced Freud and from which psychoanalysis has drawn nourishment in the past, have been transformed. The brain, for example, is now viewed as a self-organising system in which the principle of linear determinism, of straightforward cause and effect, does not apply. Can we then believe that there is a direct, linear, deterministic relationship between the experience of a depressed mother in infancy and the develop-ment of a dead mother syndrome as an adult? What is the relation between an individual's experience in infancy and early childhood and the develop-ment of psychopathology as an adult? Can these experiences in early childhood be reconstructed from the analysis of an adult?

Freud's case history of the Wolf Man (Freud, 1918) has been acknowl-edged as the paradigmatic example of psychoanalytic reconstruction. For some, it affirms the validity of psychoanalytic reconstruction; for others, it demonstrates the impossibility of reconstructing the past in psychoanalysis (Spence, 1982). However, it is clearly evident that the trauma that was reconstructed in Freud's case history, the exposure to the primal scene, is not analogous to the trauma experienced in the dead mother syndrome. In the Wolf Man the trauma consisted of an event, whereas in the dead mother syndrome the trauma consists of a prolonged absence of affective interaction. The epistemological status of these two classes of trauma is quite different. An event such as the Wolf Man's exposure to the primal scene can, potentially at least, be observed by a third party, whereas an infant or child's internal response to an emotionally unavailable mother is a private experience that cannot be confirmed by a third party, although the infant's behavioural response to a depressed mother can be observed. Direct infant observation has confirmed that by 10 months of age the emotional responsivity of the infants of depressed mothers is already organised differently from that of normal infants (Beebe *et al.*, 1997).

Direct infant observation has also confirmed the contagious effects of maternal depression on the infant. There is both behavioural and physiological evidence that differentiates infants whose mothers are depressed compared to normal mothers. For example, it has been shown that the EEG pattern of infants of depressed mothers is altered (Davidson and Fox, 1982). These infant observations would support the supposition that a depressed and emotionally unavailable mother will impact on the subsequent development of the child and contribute to the onset of psychopathology in adulthood. Critics might respond that the findings of infant research cannot be directly transposed into adult psychoanalysis and offered as a causal explanation for adult psychopathology. Some critics dismiss altogether the relevance of infant research for adult psychoanalysis, claiming as does Peter Wolff (1996) that the relation between infants of depressed mothers and adult psychopathology is nothing more than an analogy.

There is a tendency today among some psychoanalysts to deprecate Freud's belief in historical reconstruction. Freud assumed that the historical truth of experiences in childhood could be arrived at independently of the influence of the analyst. He stated that those who claim that the analyst's constructions are no more than the analyst's fantasies about the patient, derived from his own complexes, underestimate the enormous ingenuity an analyst must possess to invent a unifying explanation from such diverse sources (Freud, 1918, p. 52). The criticism to which Freud responded has now reappeared, as some analysts doubt whether there can be true historical reconstructions apart from the suggestive influence of the analyst. Those who challenge reconstruction in psychoanalysis doubt that the truth of an individual's past can ever be known. As Donald Spence (1982) and Roy Schafer (1983) claim, there is only narrative truth and not historical truth. This argument appears to be based on logic, but we should be suspicious of arguments based on logic alone, for at the beginning of this century you will recall that philosophers logically claimed that only that which is conscious deserves to be described as mental. Spence and Schaffer assert that inasmuch as history can only be known through the eyes of the observer, a reconstruction of a patient's past is not possible. An individual's history is therefore inevitably reduced to the observer's interpretation. What we do as analysts is not to discover or reconstruct the past but to construct it. If the past cannot be 'objectively' known, the analyst can only offer his own construction of those events. Therefore, interpretations based on historical reconstruction are no more than a form of the analyst's suggestion. Interpretations are part of the analyst's narrative and a 'good' interpretation merely indicates a good 'fit' between the analyst's and the patient's narrative. Roy Schafer has stated that an 'accurate' interpretation is an impossibility for the analyst; the analyst is only offering the patient an alternative 'story line', merely substituting *his* narrative for that of the patient (Schafer, 1983). The persistent influence of the affective memories of the early mother/child interaction, implicit in the dead mother syndrome, is a direct challenge to this view.

The persistent influence of early affective memories in the absence of conscious recall is given support by recent memory research. Investigations support the view that infantile amnesia is a problem of recall, not of registration (Le Doux, 1996). We know that infantile amnesia, which is the absence of declarative memory, persists until about the age of 2 1/2. But infant researchers can demonstrate that infants remember affective interactions with their caretaker (Beebe *et al.*, 1997). These memories, however, remain implicit; they are what Bollas called the 'unthought known' (Bollas, 1987). The reason for this absence of declarative memory during this period of development has been recently attributed to the slow maturation of the hippocampus. Declarative memory is mediated by the hippocampus, whereas implicit memory is mediated by different systems; neuroscientists have observed that the hippocampus is slow to mature compared to other brain structures (Le Doux, 1996).

In evaluating the truth status of childhood trauma we are touching on a subject which, in the United States, has received widespread attention in the popular press. There has been intense debate, described as 'the memory wars', regarding the truthfulness of traumatic memories of putative victims of physical and sexual abuse. There are those who believe that to question the authenticity of the memory of such abuse is an injustice to the victims. Out of this belief there arose a movement of naïve or untrained therapists who either suggest abuses when they have not occurred or accept all of the patient's fantasies as fact. Meanwhile, on the other side, there are those who believe that it is unjust to punish alleged child abusers if memory itself is so unreliable. How to distinguish memory from imagination and fantasy – an ancient philosophical problem – was, as we all know, the problem Freud faced when he recognised that in *some* instances he had mistakenly believed that a seduction had occurred when he was simply hearing his patient's Oedipal fantasy. In the case history of the Wolf Man, he makes the opposite claim: the Wolf Man's trauma was not the consequence of imagination or fantasy; the trauma was that of the memory of his exposure to an actual event – parental intercourse performed from behind. Witnessing the father entering the mother from behind intensified the Wolf Man's castration anxiety, as the position of the parental sexual act made it appear as if the father's penis vanished within the mother's vagina.

In his discussion of this case Freud presents a very balanced view concerning the truth value of traumatic memories: 'It does not necessarily follow that these previous unconscious recollections are always true. They may be; but they are often distorted from the truth, and interspersed with imaginary elements' (Freud, 1918, p. 51). Freud reconstructed the chronology of the primal scene from the child's nightmare of white wolves, which he dated to the Wolf Man's first year and a half of life. This reconstruction was buttressed by the fact that in the summer, six months from his first birthday, the Wolf Man suffered from a malaria attack which made it likely that he would be allowed to sleep in his parent's bedroom. As I have noted, the truth status of a memory of an affective interaction with the mother is of a different order. No one can question the fact that the affective memory *is* the patient's experience of the past. It is the patient's experience alone and to question the truth of it seems incoherent. Whether in fact the mother was depressed and emotionally unavailable, may or may not be confirmed by outside observers or may be confirmed by the mother herself. In one instance, when questioned by her daughter, her mother said that she was not depressed after her birth; she was 'dead'. She explained that she had no feeling for anything or anybody.

The validity of psychoanalytic reconstruction has been challenged from another direction. Some American psychoanalysts, who describe themselves as social constructivists, question the historical rootedness of the psychoanalytic process itself, asserting that it is a process created afresh in the here and now; that it is mutually constructed and contingent rather than 'caused' or determined by the patient's memories and fantasies of past experiences. This constructivist point of view again asserts that there is no validity in Freud's belief that an individual's childhood can be reconstructed, that reconstructions have no claim to historical accuracy.

Opponents of psychoanalysis have justifiably criticised psychoanalysts for offering a simplistic *post hoc* explanation of psychiatric disorders, a univocal determinism. There have been embarrassing examples of such modes of thinking, such as the unfortunate period when some psychoanalysts spoke of schizophrenogenic mothers. The term dead mother invites a similar error in that it suggests that a linear causal relationship exists between the experience of the 'dead mother' in infancy and childhood, and the subsequent development of the dead mother syndrome. It is as if the mother's emotional deadness has infected the child without any consideration of the child's resistance to infection: that there are alternate responses to an emotionally absent mother, determined by forces within the child. Although, as I noted, Green speaks of the mother imago, which is the patient's construction, Green thinks of the dead mother syndrome as metaphorically analogous to mourning; he makes it clear that the patient is responding, not to the mother's loss, but to her bereavement. 'The essential characteristic of this depression is that it takes place in the presence of the object, which is itself absorbed by a bereavement' (Green, 1983, p. 149). Both the dead mother syndrome and the dead mother complex are unquestionable responses to the mother's emotional deadness, but primary identification with the mother is only one of many alternatives.

Causality and determinism

The distinction between the *dead mother syndrome* and the *dead mother complex* illustrates the variability of individuals' responses to trauma. A total identification with the mother's affective deadness is the most pathological and malignant outcome. As I noted earlier, it is not uncommon that in the first and second year of life mothers should be depressed and emotionally unavailable to their children, and this does not necessarily lead to a primary identification with this depressed mother. Selective forces within the individual come into play that will contribute to resilience or lack of resilience. Such forces would include variations in the infant or child's cognitive capacities. Infant research has demonstrated that an infant is able to differentiate self from other, yet we attribute the blissful sense of merging with the mother to an infantile state (Modell, 1993). It is reasonable to suppose that the infant may at the same time experience simultaneously both separateness and merging. This state of affairs is analogous to Winnicott's observation of the infant accepting the paradox of the transitional object that is both created from within and presented from the outside. This suggests that the capacity to experience paradox may arise much earlier in development than we have supposed. Let us assume that there are individual variations in this capacity to accept paradox; that at some point in the first year of life some infants, and not others, will have the capacity to appreciate paradox and metaphor. Such a child may be able to play with its similarity to and difference from the mother. Even if the mother is depressed and emotionally unavailable, the outcome need not be a total or primary identification with her; the child may selectively identify with differences rather than similarities. The child may choose to become the opposite of the mother. This of course does not preclude an unconscious identification, but this state of affairs is quite different from a total or primary identification. In response to the mother's absence, the child does not attempt to recapture the mother's love through identification, but claims instead that he or she needs nothing from the mother, and anything that reminds him of the mother becomes antithetical to his sense of self. In this instance the child is not lost within the mother's psyche but constructs an individuality based on separateness. For example, instead of incorporating the mother's insensitivity to the inner state of the other, the child develops a compensatory hypersensitivity to the inner state of the other. I suspect that this state of affairs is not uncommon among those of us who have chosen to become psychoanalysts.

Hypersensitivity to one's own inner life and to the inner life of others is only one such compensatory outcome of a child's exposure to the dead mother. There are many other possible outcomes. To compensate for the fear of inner deadness, those suffering from a dead mother complex may be compelled to practice what can be described as a kind of psychological pump-priming, where they ensure their psychic aliveness by artificial means.

For example, the fear of the deadness of the self may be negated through a hypersexuality or an addiction to thrills or induced crises.

What I am proposing is that we adapt a selectionist view of development as an alternative to a linear, deterministic conception (for a similar point of view applied to the infant's perceptual and motor development, see Thelen and Smith, 1994). A selective view incorporates the belief that the brain, and by implication the mind, are 'Darwin machines' (Plotkin, 1994). Edelman, Changeux and others have proposed that evolutionary processes are operating in real time within the brain in pre-natal and post-natal development (Edelman, 1992; Changeux, 1997). The brains of identical twins differ both structurally and functionally: individuality is a literal biological fact. Everyone's brain is unique. As William Blake observed, 'A fool sees not the same tree that a wise man sees.' As every individual's brain is unique, the outcome of trauma is unpredictable. A selective process will determine the outcome of a specified environmental trauma. Just as individuals in a given species over evolutionary time will adapt uniquely to challenges presented by the physical environment, an individual, in somatic time, will adapt to the challenges of both the internal and external environments.

From this point of view, the determinants that contribute to a pathological outcome of a developmental process are beyond numeration. On a global or macroscopic level there is the question of the temperament, or mood of the individual, which is thought to be an inherited attribute. A cheerful or ebullient child will be more resilient compared to a depressive child. The obvious fact of the availability of alternative caretakers will play a crucial role in determining the outcome of a child's response to an emotionally unavailable mother. These are obvious global environmental factors. Less obvious are the variations in the child's internal cognitive capacities which I alluded to earlier, like the capacity to accept paradox and the capacity to create transformative metaphors of life experiences. These cognitive traits contribute to the child's faculty for creative fantasy and imagination. What is crucial for some individuals is the ability to construct alternative inner worlds of the imagination that will effectively remove them from the impingement of a traumatising relation with the mother.

A free-floating imagination and the ability to use metaphor to transfer meaning from one domain to another facilitate the recontextualization of memory. This process, which Freud termed *Nachträglichkeit*, may enable the individual to transcend a traumatic past (Modell, 1993). There is a significant distinction to be made between memories that are fixed and memories that have been retranscribed. There is a significant difference between those individuals who remain open to new experience and those who remain prisoners of the past.

References

Beebe, B., Lachman, F. and Jaffe, J. (1997) Mother-Infant structures and pre-symbolic self and object representations. *Psychoanalytic Dialogues.* 7: 133–82.

Bollas, C. (1987) *The Shadow of the Object.* New York: Columbia University Press.

Changeux, J.-P. (1997) *Neuronal Man.* Princeton, NJ: Princeton University Press.

Davidson, R. and Fox, N. (1982) Asymmetrical brain activity discriminates between positive versus negative affective stimuli in human infants. *Science* 218: 1235–7.

Edelman, G. (1992) *Bright Air, Brilliant Fire.* New York: Basic Books.

Freud, S. (1918) From the history of an infantile neurosis. *S. E.* 17: 51.

Green, A. (1983) The dead mother. In A. Green. *On Private Madness.* Madison, CT: International Universities Press, 1986.

Guntrip, H. (1975) My experiences of analysis with Fairbairn and Winnicott. *International Review of Psycho-Analysis,* 1975: 21–45.

Le Doux, J. (1996) *The Emotional Brain.* New York: Simon and Schuster.

Modell, A. (1993) *The Private Self.* Cambridge, MA: Harvard University Press.

Plotkin, H. (1994) *Darwin Machines.* Cambridge, MA: Harvard University Press.

Schafer, R. (1983) *The Analytic Attitude.* New York: Basic Books.

Shore, A. N. (1994). *Affect Regulation and the Origin of the Self.* Hillside, NJ: Lawrence Erlbaum.

Spence, D. (1982) *Narrative Truth and Historical Truth.* New York: Basic Books.

Stern, D. (1994) One way to build a clinically relevant baby. *Infant Mental Health Journal* 15(1): 9–25.

Thelen, E. and Smith, L. (1994) *A Dynamic Systems Approach to the Development of Cognition and Action.* Cambridge, MA: The MIT Press.

Tronick, E. (1989) Emotions and emotional communication in infants. *American Psychologist* 44: 112–19.

Wolff, P. (1996) Infant observation and psychoanalysis. *Journal of the American Psychoanalytic Association* 44(2): 369–92.

4

DEAD MOTHER, DEAD CHILD

Christopher Bollas

Antonio worked as an engineer for a construction company for about two years, but left some six months before beginning analysis. He complained that he did not comprehend why he acted in the ways that he did. He told me that he had found the construction company very challenging and thought he had done quite well there, but there were problems. He paused for some minutes, seemingly in contemplation, before resuming his account. He said that it had been 'interesting' how he had gone through a sort of crisis with his boss: he initially quite liked him, but then he believed his boss had been less than thrilled with him.

His boss had thought him unusually promising and they got off to a very good start. He was handed important projects, but then found himself disagreeing with one of the other project managers. Eventually it became clear that he withdrew into a kind of sulk in the presence of his boss and colleagues, but his employer, a hearty, well-intentioned family man, wasn't going to be deterred by his new employee's odd behaviour, and confronted him continuously over several months. Antonio thought he was always on the verge of the sack, but, as his boss informed him, although it seemed as if that was exactly what he wanted, he, the boss, was not going to accommodate him. This led to a quite profound breakthrough in which Antonio rediscovered his sense of initiative, came out of his sulk, idealised his employer, and was very content – in fact happier at work than he had ever been.

As he told me the details of this story and the tale unfolded and deepened, he gradually became less communicative. It felt like a resistance of a peculiar kind, as if he had suddenly been overcome by something. When I drew attention to anything he said, or to his silences, it lit him up and drove him to further speech; smiling, as if awakened from some distracting sleep, he would suddenly tell me in much greater detail what he had intended to discuss.

I commented on the moments when he began an hour with promise, only to withdraw into what seemed to me puzzling silences, eliciting forms of pursuit from myself. When I said this he often broke down into uncontrollable sobbing. Within a few weeks of beginning analysis Antonio, who initially seemed talkative, composed and alert, was transformed into an often mute, distraught, and lifeless looking self. It was as if 'something had come over him'. Now he entered sessions like a figure out of the *Walking Dead* films, his face drawn and expressionless, only moving into a vestige of life when I asked him what he was thinking, this ordinary question throwing him momentarily back into something of the lively self that had entered analysis.

Still, he continued to tell me about his life outside the analysis. It was with considerable disappointment that his employer had to accept Antonio's well-reasoned resignation notice. He believed it was in his best interest to undertake an advanced training course in engineering and he wished his boss and colleagues a fond farewell. He left after a very moving Christmas party, when the entire *corps de construction* toasted his future, unaware that he had no course to enter. He felt a kind of inner distillation of a powerful secret, but his sadness, forlornness, and sense of fatedness seemed absolutely real in response to his departure.

In these early months of psychoanalysis he told me in halting but considerable detail about his childhood and adolescence. He was the third of five children, three girls and two boys. His parents had lived in Sicily until he was 4, and then moved to England, where they hoped to find a better life for themselves. This did not turn out to be the case, however, as his father struggled to find work, his mother – pregnant with the next son – was depressed and distant, and he could only recall a profound shift of atmosphere within the family.

As he described Sicily, tears welled up in his eyes. Sessions drew to a halt. He would clench his face in a fisted hand squeezing himself back into composure. Then quite abruptly he would calmly describe his good memories and end many of these recollections with the statement that of course things changed in England. Antonio's manner of relating his story was as odd as the contents of the tale.

Following earlier observations and comments, I said that it felt like he was leading me up a very meaningful path saturated with feelings, but that he stopped his narrative at crucial moments to gain my increased interest in order to thwart it. He agreed. I said that we seemed to develop a sense of rapport when all of a sudden he changed or it seemed that something changed.

Once I said that his recollections seemed addictive, as if he were recharging the batteries of loss. He howled with laughter. He shook with laughter for a good three or four minutes. When he calmed down I asked what was so funny and he said that he was very amused with the way I had said that he recharged his batteries. Whatever merit there was to my interpretation – and unquestionably he felt strangely relieved at being seen – he was as responsive to my concentrated effort of speech, deriving intense pleasure from my 'delivery', even when deeply saddened.

One day, however, he sat down very calmly and looked at me unblinking. I waited for five minutes or so and then said, 'Well ...?' and he responded: 'Well ...?'. Thinking I had been misheard, I replied, 'What occurs to you?' and he said, 'What occurs to you'. It was a flat empty echo. Surprised, I said, 'Sorry?' to which he replied, 'Sorry'. I was more than a bit confused. It was rather hard to believe what was happening. I asked another question, which he then repeated, and then I told him that for some reason he was echoing me. He repeated the comment. This had never happened to me with a patient before, nor has it since, and I was unsure how to proceed. I remained silent for most of the hour, only occasionally commenting on his behaviour, and towards the end of the session I said that I did not know what his intention was, but it occurred to me that he was trying to dislodge me from my analytical position, to mock it and myself, and that something cynical and disturbing about himself seemed to be occurring. My interpretation was something like a stab in the dark. I actually did not know what to say. The experience, however, was of the death of communication; he was alive and in my presence, but it was as if the spirit of interrelating had been extinguished. I knew that I did not comprehend its meaning.

At the next session he smiled warmly, sat down, and began to talk about a new job he thought of pursuing. He made no reference to the previous session. I decided to see where he led so I said comparatively little. Nor did he mention the echoing session in the next week of treatment. By this time I felt I had colluded with something, although what that was I did not know; however, having given him what I considered sufficient time to tell me, I recollected the session and said that he had not commented on the session when he echoed my remarks. 'Oh! Oh that', he laughed. He laughed a good solid minute or so. 'That's nothing ... nothing at all.' I did not find his laughter irritating just rather odd. I did not know what to make of him, although the words 'that' and 'nothing' remained in mind, perhaps waiting their time for meaning.

He had no explanation, he said. He apologised, stated that it was not a nice thing to do to me, told me it would not happen again, and expressed his embarrassment. He went on to other things and I just listened, knowing of course that it meant something quite important, but as yet not knowing what. Something of the same curious phenomenon repeated itself, however, in that moods seemed to sweep over him, altering his mentality.

Later in this chapter we shall be considering André Green's theory of the dead mother complex, but Antonio's mirroring of me calls up an important explanation of Green's. When the mother abruptly loses her alive mothering, the child will decathect her, he argues, and substitute 'mimicry' of her for reparation. The aim of such mimicry is to 'possess the object (who one can no longer have) by becoming, not like it, but the object itself' (Green, 1983, p. 151). As we shall see, Antonio took possession of me through a form of mimicry that was abrupt and bizarre; it occurred far too early in the analysis for me to understand, thereby meeting its transferential intent – to shock me into experiencing something which had no meaning, corresponding, as we shall see, to Green's theory of action that scars the self with its meaninglessness.

Over the next year Antonio undertook several jobs and the same thing happened each time. He was exceedingly promising on interview and was definitely the 'new boy on the block' for several weeks. But when the lustre of the honeymoon period waned he would withdraw and cease to work as expected. Each time his employer would initially express some concern. Perhaps he had been expected to do too much to begin with? No, he replied, if anything the work was rather simple. Maybe he was tired; he looked pale. Yes, perhaps, he would say. A few weeks of the same would pass and his employer would call him into the office to chat. These events were strikingly similar; there was little difference between the situations. His puzzled employer would wonder what was wrong and Antonio would assure him that things would be put right. The employer would reply that time had already gone towards just that. Could he not explain in more detail what was going wrong? Tears would well in Antonio's eyes, the employer would find himself personally moved by this event. Reluctantly and with solemn exasperation the boss would tell him he had no choice but to sack him.

Quite a few sessions were spent discussing what was taking place with the employer, which I interpreted in the transference and linked to early events in his childhood. By then it had long since become quite clear that he had found his brother's birth and his mother's attentions to the rival unbearable. He retreated into a sulk that lasted his entire childhood, made worse no doubt, by the parents' apparent failure to perceive what he was doing. So far as he could make out they understood him to be quiet, shy, and serious. I said that he seemed born into new situations and enjoyed a good honeymoon with mother, but after this wore off, he expressed his anger by turning it against himself. I told him that I thought he found relief in my having seen this side of him and that it was one of the reasons he laughed so frequently when I confronted him in sessions: it was a relief to be found out. We rarely referred to the echoing session, although I told him that I thought he had shown me someone else, a hated person who was meant to be shoved aside, and that it seemed to me this was his notion of what was in store for him with me.

Every few months or so he would come to a session in a very dark mood. He would tell me he was having very strange thoughts. He was certain that people on the bus were talking about him. They found his way of sitting odd and were commenting to one another about it. Or while walking down the street he was quite certain that people reckoned that he smelled. I listened and asked him to tell me all that was on his mind during such moments, and his fantasies were elaborate, dense, and profoundly paranoid. They had one element in common. Each fantasy occurred in the context of a mood of profound aloneness and I told him that however disturbing these ideas were, they were none the less failed efforts at soothing: he needed to feel that he was the object of some interest, even if it seemed odious. In time the person they saw was, as I pointed out, the crippled part of himself, which he felt had never been cared for, and that needed attending. I said that he had been presenting me these aspects of himself for years, and showing it to employers, but no one seemed to know what to do about it.

Antonio found relief through my continual interpretations of the depressed and what seemed at the time the vengeful boy who did not know how to express his love and only knew how to turn things sour. Over the years, he found these comments useful, and he could take himself on in differing walks of life. He began dating for the first time, and although he had quite a few girlfriends, he eventually settled for one person. He retrained as a graphic designer and slowly re-entered the job market.

As we shall see, these interpretations were slightly aside from the core of his despair, so it is interesting to consider none the less why they were of use. Even if they overlooked the true cause of his anguish, they offered him an explanatory structure into which he could unconsciously project the deeper sources of his despair, and through which he could re-imagine himself and gain some true relief. In fact, however, the strange transformation of self – from ordinary thinking to bizarre mentations – came over him, as it were, from the outside like someone catching a virus. He clearly conveyed this in the way he described these states of mind and their contexts: for example, he was walking along Oxford Street when suddenly he was overcome by a strange idea, or he was riding a bus when suddenly he felt people were talking about him. I focused on the mental contents at this time, on the state that seemed to change in his mind. The mental contents in themselves were obviously of considerable interest and concern within the analysis, and revealed particular states of anxiety or depression on the day.

At first, however, their contents were reported exclusively within a paranoid context, but the paranoid milieu as exclusive narrative dissolved itself and he ceased thinking these thoughts only in this way. He would report his fantasies genuinely seeking understanding of their immediate origin.

But now and then he would tell me in darkened mood that he was having violent fantasies. He thought of punching people on the bus, or knifing people on the Underground, or blowing up buildings. When he reported such contents he would look down at the ground, hands between his legs, in a solemn rather self-executional manner. I would wait, silence would fall, and after a while I would take up the contents and ask for associations, including the day's context: what he had been doing just before such thoughts. Clearly he was not pleased about working in this manner but complied, particularly after I indicated to him my realisation that he seemed to want such thoughts to define him as monstrous. That they might mean something beyond themselves, as it were, interfered, I suggested, with his wish to see himself in a castigating universe.

Once again, my approach though useful in some respects, continued to miss what as yet I had not been able to comprehend. I did not see that his peculiar thoughts, which overcame him when in the company of fellow travellers, were like visitations of the bizarre, sweeping over him, and carrying him off from himself, just as they swept through the occasional fellow traveller, who would see a man shifted by passing thoughts into an uncomfortable frame of mind. He described occasions when he would be talking to a passenger on the bus, only to have a bad idea pass through his head, which would then end his social engagement, rendering him a kind of headstone for the departed.

Time passed, however, and the interesting contents of his thoughts diminished as they were deconstructed by the ordinary course of his free associations. In the overdetermined world of the symptomatic, if his character structure was only partially met by this process, the works of the dynamic unconscious still revealed their meanings through the free associative method. It was not difficult to see that they dramatised barely suppressed emotional reactions to precise experiences that just preceded them. So by returning to the scene of the injury and reconsidering it, he was able to put his distress into language; this intrinsically detoxified the violent nature of the fantasies and he became less disturbed. Eventually, however, it was important for him to understand why he had had so many violent thoughts, and furthermore, why he seemed to amplify them when they occurred.

His bitterness towards his parents was not unknown to him, and he knew that by adolescence he was unusually preoccupied with feeling a deep grudge against them, although in another part of his personality, he felt love and affection toward them. He knew that he was not being fair to them and that he was indulging his bitterness, but he could not stop it. Furthermore, there was simply too much odd pleasure in acting out the same scenario with his employers, and with women friends. These enactments abated with the analysis, but I still did not understand his curious celebrations of the violent thought.

I said he enjoyed startling people and we recollected his efforts to do this with me, conjuring a violent idea to see if he could nurse it along until it became horrifying: sufficient even to scare himself. He was well aware of this. I openly wondered if during his early childhood, perhaps due to the arrival of his brother that intensified his envy, he had experienced an increase in hate and his mental contents had become too violent too early. (I was thinking here of a kind of premature ego development in which the child becomes aware of his destructive feelings and ideas too soon. In his case from the age of 4.)

This made emotional sense to him. He remembered feeling that he was deeply alien and bizarre as a child, and believed he thought of himself like this when he was 6. I said that his reports of violent mental contents had had a curious feel to them, as if he were dramatising some other self, to see what it would do or say and how it would be received. I emphasised this as a dramatic act rather than a personal commission, and he agreed that these statements lacked conviction and that he was well aware of their monstrous quality as a matter of intrigue in their own right.

From this point I said that in my view he was showing me that he really did not know what to do with his violent thoughts. They fell upon him just as they fell upon me in the sessions. They were comprehensible and upon understanding vanished. But he experienced them as containing a deep essential truth about himself that surely, due to their power and authority, displaced any notions he might otherwise entertain about himself. I said that this left him feeling that he had no option but to side with the monstrous thoughts and try to make them into his own, even if he was personally and privately horrified and confused by them.

It was not difficult to hypothesise a split in his early childhood that drove a wedge between a loving and reparative self and the hating and violent self. The increment in his hate had led to too many destructive ideas, suggesting to him as a child that he was evil, an idea to which he capitulated. As his parents were good people and as he suffered no gross abuse at their hands, his hate was compounded by a destructive envy of what was good about them, his siblings, and himself that led him to dispatch loving feelings (towards others and himself) with ruthless abandon. He believed he did not deserve to thrive and whenever he embarked on a new job or started up a new relationship he ruined it by turning himself into a Richard the Third, darkening the stages of his life with brooding malevolence. In fact, however, he was desperate for someone to 'see through him' as had been the case with one of the employers and was true of course of my work with him. All this gave him hope, but in the therapy this hope was very risky indeed and on innumerable occasions he was unconsciously compelled to prove me wrong: that he was a monster and that his good feelings were only false ephemera.

As is often the case, the analyst's countertransference can be of assistance in making a clinical decision about some of the underlying truths that patients present. Antonio's violent thoughts did not alarm me. They puzzled me. I found them curiously eruptive and oddly out of place. I took that feeling to possibly mirror his own: that they just seemed to happen, as with obsessional patients who have compulsive thoughts that just seem to fall upon them come what may. But Antonio was a likeable person and I also took this to be an indication of the effect of his unconscious love of the other. He was also genuinely cooperative and truly relieved upon analytical interpretive work, and so I knew – I thought – from this that he was not as ill as he needed to be.

Looking back now, I could put it differently: the illness he carried was from somewhere else, an 'interject' not an introject. An interject is an internal object that arrives in the internal world either due to a parental projective identification, interjected into the self, or to a trauma from the real that violates the self, or both. An introject always expresses an aspect of the self's need or desire – a complex inner organisation reflecting the vicissitudes of the self's status over time – while an interject is an interruption of the self's idiom by the forceful entry of the 'outside'. Differing types of hesitation, uncertainty, blankness, and stupor reflect the presence of an interject which as the work of the other (or real) bears no internal sign of unconscious meaning: it simply 'sits' inside the self, its ideational content bounded by seizures of thought or behaviour At the time, however, all I knew was that my understanding of him was incomplete. There was no point in pushing it, I thought. I would just have to wait.

Antonio was spooked by his mental contents, however, so work could meanwhile take place in this area to some beneficial effect. His bad thoughts scared the hell out of him. The price he paid for years of childhood revenges against his parents, all of which were purely internal, was to cultivate a genre of horror fantasies that could scare him witless, although increasingly he realised that they also amused him. Or more pertinently, when he had a bad thought he would set up cinema within himself, popcorn stand included, and sell tickets to the other portions of the self which in states of carefully deployed innocence could walk into an unfolding scene of horror to their extreme fright. But as with the horror film addict, such scenes were also exciting, and of course it was a great relief to have survived.

Those for whom life is a trauma register this fact in a very particular way. When Antonio's parents moved from Sicily the entire family endured a trauma together. His father removed himself from the children, not because he wished to, but because circumstances in his new country required that he work long and hard hours. He missed his children. Antonio's mother was saddened by the move and she lost her intimate relation to Antonio; indeed her mood seemed a curious witness to the truth imposed by the event.

Antonio recollected the small village in Sicily where he spent his first four years. His father managed a small citrus collection centre and was a man of considerable repute in the village. He can remember the way his father would walk down the street, received by people who clearly respected him: he was a proud and accomplished man. His mother did not work, but she and her sisters and relations would sew, cook, talk, and enjoy the children together. Antonio's memories of the nooks and the crannies of the house, the garden, and the perimeter of the house were finely detailed.

The move to England annihilated all of this. The father could only find menial labour and his spirit was destroyed. The mother had lost her family and the village she loved. She went to work for the first time, continued to have other children, but could not find a way to re-root herself. Antonio's family moved house several times, eventually settling in a rather dismal bungalow in south-east England where they lived a joyless life, watching television, occasionally talking about Sicily, and avoiding at all costs upsetting anyone in the family. Each member seemed to be nursing a private devastation and no demands or reproaches could be made without one person or another immediately becoming grief-stricken.

An event had, in other words, profoundly altered the family. Antonio's parents collapsed along with him, in response to the event, which then assumed its priority over them, and indeed over the effect of the personal.

Event-traumatised individuals live in a rather suspended state, defined in part by the intrusion of the real into the personal, and the fascination in popular culture with the 'walking dead' – disturbed in their natural migration from the death of the body to its burial by a *natural event* (usually a sunburst, a peculiar storm, or radiation) – testifies to the distinction between the event-inspired trauma and the person-inspired trauma. Indeed, Mary Shelley's *Frankenstein* and the subsequent figures of scientifically resurrected corpses, cannily represents the position of the family aiming to recover from a deadening experience which left the family in limbo. The family tries to doctor its murdered participants back into a form of life and to some extent succeeds. Antonio's mother took a certain grim pride in the fact that they all survived, although each of the children was in his own way a kind of walking dead, a revived corpse which could exist, but whose gait was evidence of a death and depressive transformation. The transforming figures – the mother, the father, the family culture – resurrect the children in the wake of a trauma that has left them all shattered, but inevitably the act of transformation is saturated with grief. In putting the pieces of the family back together again the members cannot overcome the effect of the event and this informs their subsequent selves.

Antonio felt himself to be a reconstructed child. Devastated by the move which had wasted the family, he intended that it not be forgotten. His remembering took the form of mutating himself in the presence of the other, transforming what appeared to be an ordinary amiable relation, into a bizarre eruption that drove the other into a corner. As we shall see, however, this devastation-by-a-move proved so malignant because it, in turn, remembered an earlier devastation by movement. But we shall come to that.

Although Antonio was shattered by the family's move, the mother's pregnancy, the birth of his brother, and his mother's withdrawal from himself and his other brothers, he always knew that she loved him, as did his father, and yet he felt deeply harmed by both parents. I have pointed out that the full course of the trauma was really only achieved through his response to these events, when he personalised them through hatred of his parents, which in turn maximised the hating parts of his personality. This had a knock-on effect. He developed a monster self which subsequently began to bother and shock him. He felt possessed by evil, yet he could almost turn it on or off as he chose. If a bad thought crossed his mind, he could cast it aside one way or he could convert it into a trailer for a feature film that was soon to follow, and he could darken the self like a cinema dimming the lights to better see projected images.

He became something of a dramatist. It would be incorrect to state that his dramatisation of his early life was an hysterical action, in the sense that it was a form of reminiscence, but it is true to our understanding of what that word means, to use it obliquely to refer to his cinematics as theatre. Each dramatisation seemed to take him by surprise, but of course we know better: there was always an entrepreneurial part of the self present, ready with projector and screen, to stage a film if he so wished. The other half of him – the innocent – did not know of this self, and so he was routinely shocked by the arrival of the other side of himself, which left him shaken and forlorn. Here we can see the two stages: the arrival of a shocking event (the thoughts themselves), and the effect of such arrival upon the self (to create a sense of evil).

The child who has been disturbed by an event that too early in life sets him to hating his parents for it, casts himself into a very anguishing form of hell. The pain caused by the original trauma is exploited by the child to become his primary sense of self, and the pain displaces the open-mindedness and emotional receptivity of the child, who closes himself around anguish and manufactures internal objects to play out the rage of the distressed self. The unconscious guilt that is generated by the abuse of the actual parents, through grotesque caricature in the internal world, only makes matters worse, as the child must then seek negative *qualia* in his relation to the parent in order masochistically to impale himself upon parental presence whenever possible. The unfortunate consequence of this all too effective strategy is its success. The child hides his violence, cultivates bad parental objects, substantiates his hate by focusing only on bad moments with the parents and by negating anything good, all done so often within the schizoid realm of a false self that can appear quite superficially benign. Antonio acknowledged that so far as he could tell his parents thought he was just a bit too serious and solitary. He was quite sure that they had no idea what was going on in his mind.

Obviously, looking back on the echo session, we can see that Antonio launched his other half into the session, aiming to cause me not only an experience of the bizarre, but also to show me something that, as it were, would totally disappear in the next session. It was a transference of the purely internal world and as I did not actually live there, except as a specular other, I was in the first instance only an echo of myself. So when he echoed me, he simply kept me locked up in the internal world that is not meant to have a true engagement with the other. But of course this was the challenge. Did I see what happened? Or didn't I?

Did I experience a radical change in the atmosphere of our life together? Was I forced into being an outsider, thrown into a dissociated state, observing the world from a place of anxiety?

Antonio once used the term 'mutant' to describe himself. When he said this he rather bellowed emptiness but there was nothing humorous at all. To his pleasure the joke was only to be on himself. The word stuck in my mind, however, and it was only after some time, when we were reflecting on his early life, that I said it seemed an apt description of a self that was changed by a sudden event. As the years passed I reconsidered some patients with whom I had worked and realised that they too considered themselves mutants, people suddenly altered by a radical change that created a new and grotesque breed, but one that also often heralded a permanent change. One that could be passed down from one generation to the next, creating a separate race, like a group of vampires that live a separate life hidden under their tombstones during the day.

These people are often schizoid personalities, although I think schizo-phrenic individuals also testify to a sense within them that they have been dramatically changed by an event. The schizoid character, however, seems to recall easily the period of self mutation. The schizophrenic can only mythologise the moment of mutation, calling up extra-terrestrial forces, or actual genetic mutations, or germs in the environment, which permanently altered the self. Both none the less recall a moment of mutation when they became different, leaving them with a mutational self, which bears in its inscape, the self that existed before the trauma, the event that was traumatis-ing, the altered self, and what Winnicott (1954, p.281) termed 'the caretaker self'. Knowing they have endured a change to their personality, such individuals must call upon a certain kind of personal parenting to hold themselves together, lest their new character break out into its own form of madness. Schizoid stiffness or schizophrenic cold alarm are efforts on the part of the ego, to hold the mutational self in place.

People who feel they are mutationally changed rather than psycho-developmentally evolved convey this sense of fatedness by creating a curious atmosphere around themselves, achieved through odd gestures, idiosyncratic movements, and curious verbalisations of their states of mind, which give off the feel of an impending climactic change. Something is in the air. Some-thing may be on the verge of happening. The world is not to be taken for granted. What we think of as human must not be assumed. They have experienced a change in the self due to a change in the atmosphere of childhood – like radiation or chemical toxin that mutates the folks of the horror genre – and they not only remember this atmospheric change, but also believe it has altered them for ever.

It is not surprising that individuals like Antonio who have suffered from the events of a life are deeply wary of any subsequent change, even if it is theoretically for the better. The fear of psychoanalysis is understandable; the analytical process is the theatre for psychic change, so brings to the mind of an individual a deep fear of the harm which processes beyond the control of the self can inflict. This person has much in common with those who bear in them a knowledge of the structure of evil (see 'The structure of evil', in Bollas, 1992). This knowledge has specific characteristics. The self in distress is offered assistance by one who appears good and thus elicits trust and dependence from the distressed, but who uses the appearance of the good as a lure for a catastrophic reversal, when the distressed now finds himself at the destructive mercy of one who will turn need into a life-threatening situation. At the root of such knowledge is the experience of good and the trust one puts into the world for well-being, a belief that is radically destroyed by the other, and results in different forms of self destruction.

Although Antonio has knowledge of a structure of evil, in which the good can be seemingly presented in order to change itself into malevolence at the expense of a trusting other, he is not a walking killer – someone who identifies with the act of murder; but he feels himself to be a walking mutant, a limbo man, between life and death. What he has to his benefit is the memory of parental effort to revive him, even if parental acts of reparation were overly saturated with a grief that made the ego a depressed caretaker.

The knowledge, however, of having once been in good psychic shape as opposed to that self derived from an intervening trauma, creates in this individual a deep memory of two selves: one that can thrive, the other which destroys life. Antonio's other half is the alternative self he became under the force of circumstances and with which he is identified. In his personal relations, as in the analysis, he ruptures the world created by the good self, with a suddenly arrived mutation, that heralds the transformation of lived experience from benign to traumatic. The people in Antonio's life are forced to endure a sequence of actings out by him which has a memorable beginning, a middle and an end. It is like a happening that has turned things sour.

Towards the middle of his analysis, Antonio's comprehension of his identification with the rupturing event led to the crystallisation of new material. It became clear that he did not want to leave the structure of his transference, one that involved his repeated presentation of what André Green terms 'blank mourning' (Green, 1983, p. 146). For some time this had taken the form of his retreating into a sulk to be rescued by forms of interpretation on my part, which in turn became the object of interpretation in its own right. Now it seemed that this forlorn testimony was meant to be a presentation to me, a gift to my creativity: he would be bereft, I would transform him. The cumulative effect of this enactment, however, revealed love 'in the maternal necropolis' (ibid., p. 167) as this grief-stricken self was a kind of Sleeping Beauty to be awakened by the kiss of alive speech. It was never intended, however, to change in its structure, as the dead object was always meant to be a lure for any presumed live object in a romance of life with death.

As this became more comprehensible, Antonio also made several crucial visits home, returning to sessions after weekends with his parents. No sooner was he in the house than he felt gripped by the family atmosphere, one which he always thought was defined by the catastrophe, but one now reassessed. He told me how he witnessed his father frequently trying to help his mother sort something out – in cooking or tidying up – but that she seemed incapable of being moved to receive assistance, wedded instead to the agony arising out of the smallest of problems. In a rather sudden flash of insight Antonio wondered if perhaps the move to England had been necessitated by maternal despair with Italy, one which the father may have tried to remedy by leading the family into a promised land. He reconsidered his long-held view that the family was somehow a passive victim of the move.

At the same time I took a different view of the transference. What did it mean, I asked myself and eventually my patient, that Antonio's ruptures were of so little deep distress to the other? For however frustrating it was to his girlfriends to find him withdrawing, or to his employers, or to myself in working with him, he dosed the disappointment with an astonishing flourish of masochistic skill, transforming the other's disappointment into bewilder-ment and finally into a kind of remove. This dissociation aimed, however, to preserve the imagery of withdrawal, to prevent its eradication through the other's expression of anger. He was to make himself into a still life, a picture never to be forgotten, forever engraved on the other's mind. 'Behind the dead mother complex,' writes Green, 'behind the blank mourning for the mother, one catches a glimpse of the mad passion of which she is, and remains, the object, that renders mourning for her an impossible experience' (1983, p. 162). Behind this drama, or one should say, projected by this drama on to a transcendent screen, is a picture of passion: of a self forever forlorn, unforgettable, inconsolable. 'The subject's entire structure aims at a fundamental fantasy,' Green continues: 'to nourish the dead mother, to maintain her perpetually embalmed' (ibid., p. 162).

Antonio broke off relationships in order to pass on to the other a part of the mother's dead soul, a picture-fetish of the dead mother that becomes the love object. 'Thin husks I had known as men/Dry casques of departed locusts', wrote Pound in the Cantos, 'speaking a shell of speech .../Propped between chairs and table .../Words like the locust-shells, moved by no inner being;/A dryness calling for death.' When Antonio died before the eyes of the other he returned in their minds as an after-effect, a dryness calling for death.

The answer to the question, why was this not so disturbing, began to form itself. Had Antonio been too off-putting he would have been dismissed and hate aroused in the other would have mitigated the other's guilt or remorse; but by dissociating self and other from his mutational moment, he froze self and other before a painting, at an exhibit formed by the absent object, and one far too puzzling to evoke customary rage.

It is important to bear in mind a difference between mutational and developmental change. The individual who is altered by trauma transforms this deficit into the structure of a wish and henceforth seeks dramatic events as the medium of self transformation. The person who has simply evolved, disseminating the idiom through its choices of object, gets on with the quiet aspects of this rather remarkable unravelling. Such an individual finds the peace, solitude, contemplativeness, quiet urgency, conflictual density, and subtle shifting of an analysis almost like a true home for the psyche-soma, while the mutational soul finds its atmosphere Arcadian and therefore frustrating.

Those who have suffered the trauma of an event cannot successfully identify the personal with the structure of an event, because although it involves people, it is beyond the purely psychical. It does not have an originating subjectivity, a locale within the self or the other. It is beyond the person and yet person-created. The child who has been mutated by the event develops an attachment, therefore, to the nature of mutational eventfulness rather than to the presence of the other. They seek malignant events like some seek relations with people.

But is the dead mother's death not a personal death? How could it be regarded as an event from the real?

Depression often descends upon selves. Although it has a psychic origin and an unconscious meaning, it may overcome the self the way a virus grips the soma. The kind of death suffered by the mother in the dead mother complex is also dead as a psychic event at the time of its occurrence; although it has meaning, the meaning is lost to the mother experiencing it. While despair, sadness, or frustration sweeps into the psyche of all mothers ('the certain hour of maternal sorrow', Eliot), troubling them to think themselves through the moods, the dead mother refuses her own moods, killing off contact with the processes of inner life. As she dissociates herself from her affects, she stands as a continually stricken witness to the unforeseen misfortunes imposed upon her by lived experience and its after-effects. After-effects are not for her; she is dead to them.

Returning from one of his home visits Antonio described his mother's response to a failed family outing. They had intended to walk in a park but it had rained and the father and another sibling had suggested going to a museum instead. The mother disowned this solution, instead dying with the turn of events, transformed into a stricken being. Antonio was stunned by the realisation that he felt, ever so briefly, an erotic response to his mother's collapse, as if she were offering herself to the gods: a sacrificial gift ... the newly dead to the long since dead.

Of course it may be argued that each and every one of us knows the experience of mutation. Certainly we can reflect upon significant events that had an effect upon us and we know something of the mutational moment, when we are different due to a precise experience. But the traumatised person has experienced a process of continuous radical shifting from his idiom to something else and his self is derived from an event and its structure. There is a special sense of the self as a born again monster, one killed and then resurrected in a new form, mutated by the trauma, which indeed becomes part of the newly created visage.

If the event is *Nachträglichkeit*, in the case of Antonio, an evocation of the death of the mother, then becoming the something else is an act of secret devotion to the mother's dead body.

A split in the self is established very early in childhood. The individual has a sense of the old or true self which once existed. Then there is the false or mutant self, derived from force of circumstance. That ordinary intrapsychic object relation between the internal *I* and the *you* that derives out of the natural internalisation of the fundamental relational structure between self and other, is transformed by its grotesque double, one in which the *I* is the vestige of a former true-self structure – that is it is the place of the observant consciousness – but now relating to a *you* that is a new creature. This new creature gazed upon from a dissociated *I* bears *its* own grudge, as it was created out of the unnatural, 'Frankensteined' by the science of events which no human other could successfully manage or repair.

If the malignant event is the descent of death into the mother, who offers it as her passion, then the child of such circumstance may auto-eroticise his own dissociation: out of his death and the sprung double – from old self to bizarre new self – arrives a love relation.

The individual traumatised by the event, then, believes that he or she is parented by something other than the human, by the molecularity of accidents committed in the presence of others but not intended by them. Such people are surprises. They do not have an inner harmony, or live within the generative illusion of understanding (of self and other) but instead regard with positive fright their inner life as an event that displaces their observant interest. Antonio, for example, could not entertain a passing thought – such as an aggressive fantasy or a sexual wish – without believing that this inner content was on the verge of overpowering him and becoming an event in the real. Sitting in the Underground looking at an attractive woman the thought would cross his mind that he was going to go over to her and touch her breast. This thought seemed a dare. It was as if his unconscious were speaking to him thus: 'Ah, you complacent idiot. You think you are master of your own house, do you? Well, you are about to be overpowered.' Antonio would break into a sweat, tense his body, grip himself, and look for the first place of exit. That is, unless he could laugh. If he could laugh his haunting laugh he could unconsciously identify with the power of the unconscious to unseat him and find solace, as if he were replying: 'Yes of course you can get me to go over there and touch her breast, indeed to french-kiss her, and then fuck her in front of everyone. What a scene that would be, huh!', whereupon he would imagine the shocked look in the eyes of the other passengers, and this would then be like a kind of practical joke. He could triumph over his anxiety by laughing.

When this occurred he would have to laugh, but knowing how odd this could look, he would put his hand over his mouth so as to control the obvious signs of a guffaw. But he knew that his laughter was visible. So he would close his eyes and rock slightly, trying to indicate that whatever was amusing him was a spontaneous internal event and had nothing whatever to do with the people around him. This was the best he could do in an otherwise acutely embarrassing moment. Although the laugh ended his conviction that he would act out the event, none the less his oddity gave rise to a recognition that he looked bizarre to the others, and this confirmed his view that he was a mutant. Indeed we may see how his conviction that he would become prey to an acting out – transformed from the psychic content to the actual event – mirrored his early life history and bizarrely recreated him according to the unnatural. Thus each and every day of his life he was reborn by the event.

On other occasions, however, he would suddenly stop being charming and step into a morbid state of self, dead of face. Fellow travellers, he could see, were quite stunned by this sudden reversal of social fortune. It looked, he reckoned, as if something unforeseen had happened to him. Either way, he believed that he left people with a haunting picture of him, which in time we understood to be a kind of love bracelet.

The individual lives now outside himself, considering himself an outsider. Thrown into the outside by the structure of events, he now is *there* in the place where *it* happened, and in that place he observes the self that is mutilated by the course of events. He carries the structure of this phenomenon within himself. Sometimes Antonio would startle another person and bring about a dissociated moment. Sitting opposite a passenger on the train, his nose in a book, he would speak clearly but seemingly from nowhere, saying something that seemed to have nothing to do with the appropriateness of the occasion. 'Your socks are rather nice', he would say to a fellow passenger as the train whisked by the familiar places. The passenger rarely answered, so disembodied was the comment. I can only surmise that the passenger may have wondered if, in fact, he truly heard what he heard. But I reckon he knew that Antonio had in fact spoken these words and that furthermore he was presaging the possibility of an odd moment. Antonio would note the discomfort aroused in the passenger. He would cross his legs suddenly or bustle about in his briefcase. After a few minutes, the passenger might go and sit elsewhere. The point is that he had introduced a dissociative factor in an otherwise ordinary situation, interrupting the other's harmonic relation to themselves as an object, throwing them outside the internal place, into looking at the actual other, looking at themselves through the imagined (and presumably mad) eyes of the other, now quite uneasy about what would happen. He traumatised the other in the way he himself had experienced the traumatic. A human being was present. But the human being had become either the author or the associate of the eventful-as-disturbance, which now seemed beyond human comprehension and human resolution. The shudder that runs through the body of the unsuspecting bears momentarily the effect of a micro-trauma, a small token of the mutational self's being.

What event had destroyed the mother? Where did it come from? What was its character?

Antonio was an Iago–Othello all to himself, presenting the 'beast with two backs' to the other, witnessing the auto-erotic primal scene: the happening between forces of intercourse taking place solely within the self. How would an Oedipus enter this space? Where is the point of entrance? Was the event that deadened the mother from the outside, or, did it arise from the inside, from some unknown and unperceived place?

A schizoid person like Antonio who is alone most of his life shunning close or collegial relations with others naturally increases the power of the internal voice, that subvocal medium through which we utter our thoughts and talk to the self. The inner voice lies between the dream – a more deeply and purely internal phenomenon, and speech – when the subject enters the interpersonal world through utterance. The inner voice receives the imagery and textures that derive from dream objects but also imagines social encounters in which one must make the self sensible to the other. It is a kind of messenger from the world of dreams to the domain of speech, and from the society of actual others to the culture of pure wish.

Demons were originally understood to be intermediaries between the divine and the mortal, spirits that passed freely from one domain to the other, performing a valued function. By transporting the texture of his inner dialogues into social space Antonio transferred his inner world into the outer world unconsciously aiming to put before the other the nature of what he found so disconcerting. We cannot blame the fellow passengers on the train for their discomfort with his disembodied utterances; he was putting them in that internal space in which he lives as the constant recipient of such shocking commands.

Was the mother deadened by a nightmare? A dream from which she recoiled, disappearing from life and its after-effects?

This inversion of a self, in which the inner world of self and object representations is oddly externalised, reverses and yet expresses the effect of the traumatic upon a self. The move which dislodged Antonio from his unselfconscious personal development forced him to be prematurely aware of his inner objects and in turn to associate these mangled selves and objects with the outcome of the move. They were internal mutants which he felt had to be transferred back into the external world from where they came: shoved back into the real.

We think of psycho-development as evolving stages of mental tasks, each incorporating the accomplishments of the prior challenges that constitute a maturing of the self as it encounters increasing complexity in the world. Each stage is marked by a feature of its rite of passage and the oral, anal, phallic and genital stages all indicate complex challenges in the negotiation of body change and intersubjective engagements. Each stage re-invents the self's interests and desires as well as its anxieties and depressions. But ordinary people also think of life as marked by important events that challenge or inspire one to differ from former selves and to inaugurate new perspectives. Thus most of us learn from experience and are continually informed by our life.

For someone like Antonio, however, life is not marked by such stages. There is no history of seminal moments. Instead all of life seems to have been arrested and stamped by one event that stops any further psychic development. Psychoanalytic treatment, by its very nature, challenges the stasis of such a person as the associative process, and the analyst's off-beat interpretations vary the patient's frozen accounts and destabilize what has become a frozen narrative. The transference returns the self to its arrest in time and from there, needs and desires arise that enliven a moribund soul. Antonio did change, very, very, slowly, over eight years and he did come to a path of psychic development which now and then he travelled, occasionally jumping off for a moment's self arrest – but then returning to take part in the spice of life.

Green writes:

> The transformation in the psychical life, at the moment of the mother's sudden bereavement when she has become abruptly detached from her infant is experienced by the child as a catastrophe; because, without any warning signal, love has been lost at one blow.
>
> (Green, 1983, p. 150)

It was this loss, in one blow, that Antonio presented to me in the transference in the early years of our work; a loss that took the form of a sudden change of his mood, without warning, indeed without any apparent meaningful affective context to himself. His own transformed moods seemed not to be of his own making. And although he acted these blows upon the other, more often and more pertinently, he enacted maternal detachment, by suddenly acting out an apparent passing idea, and abandoning any sentient effort to comprehend himself in the moment of the enactment.

When Antonio fell in love with Melinda he celebrated the moment of un-enactment, a spell, when he felt the sudden arrival of the catastrophe from within, but he 'stuffed it'. Days passed and it remained un-enacted. He recalled a time some ten years earlier, with Gretchen, whom he loved very much and who was totally besotted with him. They had spent the day walking along the Thames and were having a coffee, before heading home for dinner, when suddenly his entire self state changed. 'What is the matter?'

she wondered. 'Nothing', he replied. To each query, he replied 'Nothing'. In one hour the relationship, which had been building promisingly for over one year, was destroyed. He said he wasn't feeling well, told her he needed to go home, and he left her in the cafe. He refused to answer her phone calls, did not open her letters, and months passed. This pattern was enacted repeatedly. And although of course she felt abandoned, the abruptness released by Antonio was for him a form of self abandonment, a 'meaningless' indifference to his own fate. Actions committed by the self seemed not to be of the self. They were the work of some other. And in this respect, such an odd attitude – customarily seen in psychoanalysis as the split-off portion of the personality (correct in some ways) – was in fact a recollection of an early fact of his life.

The catastrophe of abrupt detachment, argues Green, 'constitutes a premature disillusionment and ... carries in its wake, besides the loss of love, the loss of *meaning*, for the baby disposes of no explication to account for what has happened' (Green, 1983, p. 150). By removing himself without explanation, Antonio presented a catastrophe that bore no meaning either to Gretchen or to himself. Instead he succumbed to the very event he unleashed, following its logic, turning the stunning effect into the stunned self. As Green argues, the child de-cathects the maternal object and forms 'unconscious identification with the dead mother' (1983, p.150); in Antonio's case, he follows the event which he enacts and derives his character from it.

And in the period of separation from Gretchen? The character of this isolation? Let us read Green:

> Arrested in their capacity to love, subjects who are under the empire of the dead mother can only aspire to autonomy. Sharing remains forbidden to them. Thus, solitude, which was a situation creating anxiety and to be avoided, changes sign. From negative it becomes positive. Having previously been shunned, it is now sought after. The subject nestles into it. He becomes his own mother, but remains prisoner to her economy of survival. He thinks he has got rid of his dead mother. In fact, she only leaves him in peace in the measure that she herself is left in peace. As long as there is no candidate to the succession, she can well let her child survive, certain to be the only one to possess this inaccessible love.
>
> (Green, 1983, p. 156)

We may see how the strange contentment that came over Antonio during his enactments, especially in the transference, dulled what he would otherwise have imagined to be an exceedingly irritating effect. Instead the auto-erotic theatre of this love relation pulled its punches, he curled into himself, mother to his mother, other to himself, in the beginning his end, in the end his beginning.

Solitude *changes sign* – from negative to positive. This changing of the sign is part of Antonio's transference. The transference serves a sign function, rather than a symbolic meaning, one of the reasons why it is so curiously empty of meaning, yet powerful as an emptiness.

> 'That's nothing … nothing at all.'
> Nothing?
> Nothing will come of nothing.
> A no-thing.

A nothing brought into the midst of filiation. Think of *Lear*, a nothing carried by a daughter to her father in his departure from rule. Abruptness giving birth to catastrophe. And the mother: where is she to be found in the play? Perhaps recollected in the change of sign from the positive to the negative which was meant to be positive; a breach created between father and daughter, to commemorate what? The daughter's love of the father? Or memory between them of maternal absence, celebrated in the abrupt catastrophe: sudden decathexis of love. (Lear: 'We/Have no such daughter … nor shall ever see/That face of hers again.') And whose face has not appeared in the play? Whose presence is virtually unmentioned? Whose name signifies the eradicated? Perhaps, however, maternal abandonment can only announce itself in pure absence of representation, a sign that moves as an effect through the other who shall never know it, only act it.

Antonio's 'nothings' were the verbal sign of maternal absence, born upon the mood of catastrophic departure.

We may now look back on the view that it was the move at age 4 which was the sole cause of Antonio's mutation. In his repetition of love followed by radical de-cathexis Antonio demonstrates the disappearance of love from the self, leaving either a mordant presence, or, after sudden withdrawal, a totalising absence: compelling the abandoned to retrospectively assume that signs of love and affection were only appearances. The move from Sicily is engraved in Antonio's mind partly because it is memorable and partly because the family recollected the traumatic effects of the mother's de-cathexes by leaving the country. The family (mother included) could now give location to this trauma and safely grieve the loss. No one was held to blame. No one was responsible. The move, like Lear's apparently wise retirement, released the 'no-thing' born in human character, now externalised into the collective of man.

The wave of depression. The sudden loss of cathexis, of love invested in the child. What dies in Lear, as died in Antonio's mother, is love unaffected by passing moods, shifting circumstances, quirks of character. A self is overcome by 'x', forced out of its love. Antonio's sudden departures recollected maternal de-cathexis, but the dissociation precipitated by this catastrophe allowed the infant a backward glance, catching a glimpse of the falling hands, enough to find in this maternal departure an erotic distillation: the tug of love crystallised by the vanishing. As Antonio withdrew into 'born again' narcissism, deriving out of the dead mother complex, self-love is fixation on reaching for the dying love object. Her laugh is not the giggle of the mother at play in peek-a-boo, but the haunting bellow of a ghost who leaves the abandoned with a lifelong riddle to haunt the self. Antonio's sobbing would often follow prolonged, unreal, laughter. The belchings of death.

In the later years of the analysis, I found a certain line of comment increasingly meaningful. 'You were tempted to withdraw from Gretchen (his girlfriend) to see if the catastrophe of withdrawal is real', I told him. 'It is all too real', I added, 'so real as to be beyond belief and therefore – you hope – in the world only of bad dreams'. I said that I thought he wanted to test it again and again, to try to make it only a nasty turn of events, and not something that came out of the real to affect him.

The passing of time, and the fact that he was now in his late thirties, assisted the line of thought: to continue would sustain proof that we are really alive, not figments of our imagination, that we can really suffer the consequences of our decisions and that our lives really are affected. Really.

When I spoke to him like this from where did I speak? In the textures of dreams and associations? In the opaque house of memory's mirrors? In the opera house of object relations?

No.

I spoke from a place into which maternal love vanished, from the rim of dreamland, psychic life, and its object relations, a border from which we came and to which we shall return, the place of the frame from which a type of perspective is achieved. I was outside the scene, outside the transference, outside the analysis and it was from there that I could speak to him and see his recognition of a need to speak to the other on that border. In the oddest of possible ways, by speaking from the outside, I gradually put Antonio back into life itself, a necessity forced upon me from communiqués transmitted from the strange country we call transference and countertransference.

> And as imagination bodies forth
> The form of things unknown, the poet's pen
> Turns them to shapes, and gives to aery nothing
> A local habitation and name.
>
> (*A Midsummer Night's Dream*)

References

Bollas, C. (1992) *Being a Character*. London: Free Association Books.

Green, A. (1983) The dead mother. In *On Private Madness*, London: Hogarth Press and the Institute of Psychoanalysis, 1986.

Winnicott, D. W. (1954) Metapsychological and clinical aspects of regression within the psycho-analytical set-up. In *Collected Papers: Through Paediatrics to Psychoanalysis* London: Hogarth Press and the Institute of Psycho-Analysis.

5

THE UNDEAD

Necromancy and the inner world

Jed Sekoff

In the parlour

I am looking at a photograph. It carries the signs we have come to recognise as meaning 'from the past'. Sepia tones, clothes from another era, and a certain pose – somehow formal, stern, a bit distant. It is a pose common in early photographs, stemming from the need to keep still for the long exposure; or was there a certain gravity associated with the task? In any case, the image before me in London's National Portrait Gallery is a photograph of a family. The small child in the overstuffed chair lacks the aggressive face of a modern child, no squirming away or making fun. Indeed, the child looks asleep ... until it hits you. That fully dressed, posed–for–a–portrait child, is dead.

In the early years of photography, the surge of new processes (daguerreotype, calotype, gelatin emulsion) was matched by a rush of new subjects: travel sites, war reportage, pornography, police files, and by the 1860s, millions of family portraits. The poet Elizabeth Barret wrote, 'I would rather have such a memorial of the one I dearly loved, than the noblest artist's work ever produced' (1843; in Upton, 1976, p. 10). Photographs of the dead would become a staple of the time, placed on gravestone, mantlepiece, or in the family album – the deceased often posed among family and friends. A memorial is a form of memory, or rather it is a grievance against memory; it is a plea, a tonic to counter memory's propensity to fade. Susan Sontag noted that 'photographs are not so much an instrument of memory as an invention of it or a replacement' (Sontag, 1977). We photograph something that we hope to hold onto, 'to catch in our hands'. Yet how do we catch hold of death?

Looking may be a way of capturing that which cannot be held. Wish, phantasy, imagination, and memory have a common root in the eye's grasp at our elusive world. They are second looks at the spot where something was, but now no longer is. And what better second look than a photograph that captures an instant of time, a frozen moment that offers the possibility of holding time in our hands. It is claimed – perhaps apocryphally – that certain tribal peoples fear the photograph will 'steal their souls'. (Reportedly, photographers have been viewed as 'shadow catchers' and 'face peelers'.) Is this such a preposterous idea? The photographic image collects power as well as light. A captured instant interrupts the flow of time. Looking may now be gathered, collected, catalogued. A dead face lives on. Marina Warner (1995) has suggested that our laughter at the primitive fear of the camera may disguise our own craving for the magical power of the image, an expression of our wish for a means to dominate an other. Then again, perhaps it is ourselves we hope to dominate, to fool time, to trick death, to resist the relentless movement of the world.

Feared or pursued, the photograph marks a boundary. Looking at a photograph places us at the edge of a certain time. Neither the moment before or after. Yet, this singular moment, ever present, ever still, evokes a boundless space, alive, in motion. The dead are somehow conjured into life. And yet again, this very magic makes their death all the more certain; our loss stares us in the face. We might better describe the boundless boundary of the photographic image as a peculiar frontier – 'a region that forms the margins of settled territory' (Merrian-Webster, 1989) – where the flora and fauna of the past, present, and future are captured in one compact space. The imago, the psychic representation, the introject, the object, are among the names that psychoanalysis gives to the 'image-inings' that occupy this border land. Let us enter this frontier with a clinical story.

When Nina P. was about 9 years old, she began to visit cemeteries with her mother. These were not visits to dead relatives, or historical forays, nor a search for quiet in a busy city; they were on a photographic expedition. Her mother was an accomplished photographer, and her dominant subject of that time was her daughter, posed nude in graveyards atop the headstones. Several years into Nina's treatment with me, her mother mounted an exhibition of these works. There was a bit of controversy surrounding the images: twenty-plus years on, nude children were no longer considered frolicking innocents. Suspicions of exploitation and abuse were in the air, but Nina, now 32, was pleased with the photos. She liked the way she looked, how pretty she seemed. She remembered how good it felt to be the centre of her mother's attention. The graveyard seemed just a backdrop, a little spooky, also a bit of fun, what with the two of them sneaking over the walls to take the pictures. She had felt alive, alive in her mother's eyes.

Unfortunately, while the cemetery had given her no nightmares, Nina had come to feel terribly haunted. At age 14, soon after her mother stopped photographing her, she began 'coming apart at the seams'. Her body was 'no longer beautiful, I used to wonder if that was why she stopped the pictures'. Nina got 'funny about food', that is, some foods seemed safe, but others might be contaminated. There was also the problem of how much food one could take in or leave inside. Worse, she began to experience overwhelming anxiety states and dreaded 'blue feelings', painful depressive states that have plagued her on and off ever since. At 30, now a married woman, having moved with her husband to a city far from home, she began to feel an all too familiar 'unravelling'. She had seen an analyst for much of her life: he 'steadied me out', 'lifted me out of my slides'. Now, once again, she took refuge in an analytic relationship, quickly taking to her work with me. Yet, once again, her feelings of relief proved ephemeral, fading rapidly, sometimes a few hours, sometimes just a few minutes after finding help and sustenance.

What she was able to sustain, to keep in view as it were, was an image of her mother. Mother was never far from her thoughts. Each night before sleep they spoke by phone, each awakening brought their morning call. Perhaps this was simply closeness: they shared ideas and problems, agreed on dish patterns and decorating styles, they even wrote letters to each other's dolls. Still, if this was intimacy, it was a demanding one, rigid and confining. Few actions could be contemplated independent of her mother's attitudes, preferences, or criticisms. Mother's 'rules' were as strict as any industrial specification, things were either right or unforgivable. On occasions, actually, when she thought about it, almost every night, Nina considered not calling home; she was tired, her husband needed time, she didn't quite feel like it. And in the mornings she sometimes awoke hopeful, ready for her own day, until she remembered the call to come, and with it the dark atmosphere of her mother's tales of woe.

There seemed in fact to be several different mothers to cope with. There was the comforting mother, the one to tell anxieties and troubles to (though Nina noticed her own concerns seemed to pale in the face of mother's urgencies). There was the mother who seemed to treat Nina as a dumping ground, an external rendition of the 'toilet-breast' described by Meltzer. And then there was a more shadowy figure, not quite the same as the mother on the other end of the phone, but a presence inside her mind, an 'inner mom' who Nina 'bumped into' at every turn.

Of course, the psychoanalytic process invites such shadows out from the wings. Nina began to describe a sequence, a scene that went something like this: she would become aware of feeling good or unencumbered, and then, in an instant, as if that very awareness propelled what was to come, she began to 'slide downward'. As she 'fell', she caught glimpses of her mother: she 'saw' mother jumping off a bridge or lying injured on the ground, or shouting in a voice that was angry, unforgiving, and cruel. Nina was startled by these images, by how close at hand they were, by how powerfully she felt them. Yet an image is an engine of ambiguity. On the one hand, the immediacy of an image, its sensuous connection to both perception and desire evokes a fullness, a certitude of meaning. On the other, without an anchoring narrative, images drift on: the photograph of a dead child does not tell us if he was wanted or resented, if she was loving or churlish or happy. We are called upon to infuse our imaginings with meaning, and so Nina struggled to understand what she was 'seeing'. We began to explore the varied ways this image of a fallen, injured, or angry mother inhabited her daily life. The constant pressure on her chest – 'like a piano on top of me' – began to feel less a heart problem, more like another falling away from feeling good. The panic she felt during an evening out, or a walk with friends, appeared less as a breakdown, more like a measure of how far she had dared travel away from her 'inside mom'. Her fears of being poisoned by errant kitchen chemicals or food gone bad raised the question of a vengeance being exacted from within. Far from settling matters, these alternate constructions upset a delicate balance that her symptoms had provided. She felt a dizzying loss of certainty, and an intense pain at betraying versions of herself that she and others had come to rely on. The dutiful daughter, the special child, the suffering adult were giving way. Loyalty now seemed linked with fear. Specialness masked a form of submission. And suffering too, no longer seemed a fate she could gallantly endure or share.

Roland Barthes argued that to understand an image, one must look for its 'sting'; that is to say, images are punctuated by 'sensitive points' which elaborate, capture, and cast the meaning embedded in the image. Barthes named these guiding stings the 'punctum' (Barthes, 1981). For Freud, phantasies, symptoms, and dreams could be seen to have 'punctums', but he conceived these punctuation marks on the order of a photograph of someone holding a photograph of someone holding a photograph – that is, the navel of our dreams, the wishes embedded within our phantasies, or the conflict underlying our symptoms, are points of perpetual regression; more than any other psychical points, they always lead to something more.

The 'mother' lying on the ground in Nina's phantasies proved such a 'punctum'. Nina recalled mother's bouts of depression: dark, brooding, vegetative states that mother ministered with alcohol, pills, and a daughter to pour out her heart to. She remembered the air in the house, close and still, where mother's rule of open bedroom doors did not bring fresh air but blocked any whiff of privacy. And she strained to remember any voicing of her own anger, or any complaint – conflicts quelled by mother's headaches and heartaches.

Secrets also emerged. Her father's homosexuality for one. The bitter gulf between her parents was cloaked in something forbidden, something unspoken, and she drew that silence tight around her. Another silence shrouded the maternal grandmother she never knew. She was an imposing woman, cold and cruel, whose 'riding accident' was the family encryption for an apparent suicide. Mother, her inner mother, seemed surrounded by secrets that dared not be breached.

Barthes wrote that the photograph's 'punctum' is 'that accident that pricks me (but also bruises me, is poignant to me)' (1981, p. 27). Nina's image of her mother falling was a poignant bruise that pointed her, as if by accident (at least an accident of the Freudian kind) to a realm beyond recovered memory or revealed secrets. She began to notice that the image was not inhabited solely by her mother. She saw ('it's too horrible to tell') someone pushing her mother down, kicking the fallen body, someone yelling and screaming back, and she knew this someone was herself ....

In the same year and in the same city that Barthes wrote his *Camera Lucida*, another French writer contemplated imagoes that have been pierced, marked, wounded. The psychoanalyst André Green wrote of a kind of suffering, in which

all seems to have ended, as with the disappearance of ancient civilizations, the cause of which is sought in vain by historians, who make the hypothesis of an earthquake to explain the destruction of palace, temple, edifices and dwellings, of which nothing is left but ruins.

(Green, 1983, p. 150)

This depressive Pompeii he named the dead mother complex, a psychic ruin that seizes hold of the subject in such a way that all vitality and life becomes frozen, where 'in fact it becomes forbidden ... to be.' (ibid., p. 152). Coincidentally, Green points to the photographic image, to illustrate this seizure of vitality. One looks at the photos of a young baby: gay, lively, interested, compared to later snapshots where the initial happiness has drained away. With this look, and through a series of complex, richly elaborated ideas, Green points us to the 'punctum' of a particular analytic subject. A depressive, a fellow sufferer to be sure, but one with a particular adhesion to his inner world. In this image-inary landscape, a maternal imago reigns, 'a thousand headed hydra', jealous of rivals, insulated from experience, and with whom the subject remains entombed, frozen and distanced from an authentic life in the world.

On one level, Green is describing a particular pattern of pathological organisation. He charts the psychic reverberations of a child attempting to enliven a depressed, bereft, or absent mother. This resuscitation becomes the life task of the subject, accomplished through a series of manoeuvres (identification with the object, compulsive mentation, intense sexual rivalry with the object's others, auto-erotic retreat – to name but a few) that sustain a precarious link to the depleted other. At another level, Green is elaborating his project of theorising absence as a fundamental property of psychical life. Absence, blankness, emptiness, negative narcissism, white anxiety, psychical holes, non-being ... non-breast ... non-integration ... non-object ... nothingness ... these are the words, the palette of Green's epistemology of the negative.

Green opens his essay on the dead mother claiming that modern psychoanalysis is founded on the question of mourning. He goes on to chart a territory at the frontier of loss, entering a terrain where the tendency of psychic structure is to dissolve towards, revolve around, and adhere to nothingness. Certain patients, or better, certain psychical constellations, come to revolve around the proposition that 'all I have got is what I have not got'. This negative presence becomes the gravity of a psychic life founded upon loss. In this line of thought, Green joins Wilfred Bion and D. W. Winnicott as the explorers par excellence of what might be called the *negative sublime*. According to Merriam-Webster, the sublime is a beauty that inspires awe, that is to say it is a quality of an object that evokes both reverence and dread. For Green, Bion, and Winnicott the absent other marks the place, names the conditions which allow thought, being, or vitality to move forward; or inversely, becomes the graveyard of the subject, where attacks on linking (negative K) (Bion, 1959), unintegration (Winnicott, 1963), or madness (Green, 1986c) reign. In essence, the dead mother defines a kind of psychoanalysis, a psychoanalysis offered as an engagement with the 'terrible beauty' of our absences.[1]

Taking up this engagement alongside Green, we come to recognise absence as nuanced, complex, paradoxical. Absence may seize hold of us, shadow us, propel us toward oblivion, yet, absence is also constitutive, creative, a necessary condition for a vital and alive psychic life: 'Absence is an intermediary situation between presence (as far as intrusion) and loss (as far as annihilation)' (Green, 1986a, p. 50). 'In this context, absence does not mean loss, but potential presence' (Green, 1986b, p. 293).

We are reminded of the paradoxical Freud of mourning and melancholia, where what is to be forgotten must first be remembered, and where remembering is a kind of forgetting (a way of letting go). From this vantage point, absence is in opposition to the black and white space of emptiness, negativity, blank mourning, non-being, nothingness (Freud, 1917).

To constitute absence may be among our most vital tasks. For Bion, thought, love, and transformation exist only in relation to their negatives. The absent (to be without memory or desire) is a call to the potential emergence of the positive. Winnicott treasured the place not to be communicated, the solitude that allows self-emergence, and the destructiveness ('ruthlessness') that embodies the other as separate and apart from ourselves. For his part, Green elevates absence to a form of creative structure; an 'effacement' of the primary object allows a 'framing structure' for the ego to develop (a structure that shelters the negative hallucination of the mother). The potential space created within this 'frame' allows a subjectivity to emerge, with its vital affects and thoughts intact. By way of negative demonstration, he depicts the dead mother as never absent, overfilling an inadequate psychic space. In place of a protective envelope harbouring the subject, we find an ego shorn of its backdrop, and therefore floating unhinged, anchored only by the weight of its damaged objects. Nothing can truly enter this dense space, and nothing can truly emerge from it. The capacity to efface the other, to constitute absence, is our means of overcoming the stasis of repetition. Only absence allows new thought and fresh experience.

Green informs us that the dead mother complex is a revelation of the transference. Indeed, Nina elaborated the transference elements Green describes – an intense attachment to the analysis more than the analyst (though I have found this variable in other patients), and a reverberation between three positions: the fantasy of the primal scene, the Oedipus complex, and a 'blank mourning' for the dead mother. Green is clear: the struggle with loss does not preclude the sexual and aggressive phantasms of psychic reality. On the contrary, the pull of the dead mother sets these elements afire. What Green fails to pursue are the reverberations of the countertransference. If he hints at such attention in his model of technique (an alive analyst, placing his mind and affects in the service of a vital, transitional space), he neglects the implications for the transference–countertransference matrix of a psychic organisation founded upon a refusal to separate from the common body of an entombed love. Green elsewhere describes the analytic object as 'neither on the patient's side nor on the analyst's, but in the meeting of these two communications in the potential space that lies between them' (1986a, p. 48). Yet, the common body of the dead mother complex elaborates an object that is less between two subjects, than within each of their skins. At any one time in Nina's treatment, either of us might occupy the terrain of the dead other or of the captive self, the yearning subject or the frozen object. It proved imperative to be attentive to these psychical movements lest the stasis binding Nina remain mis-recognised as a one-dimensional process, rather than as the mutual construction of a beckoning object and a responsive subject.

Green postulates that it is the incapacity to efface the primary object that undermines the establishment of a framing structure for the ego. Rather than establishing representations of the mother within the mind, a fusion within a joint necropolis is shakily established. The analytic work must be balanced between a project of representing absence and offering a framing structure of its own, a psychic envelope (Anzieu, 1990) constituted through the homologues of the analytic object. Only by living under, within, and between the skin (and skin-ego) of the analytic couple may an alternative to the grim offerings of the dead mother be sought.

All this should remind us that the call of the dead mother is not simply a siren's song. Within her tight embrace the entombed child finds solace, a shelter that offers the certainties of death over the vagaries of life. This is her magical bequest: relief from the anxieties of freedom through submission to a powerful other; sustenance of the omnipotence of holding the life of another in one's hands; disguise of aggressive intent hidden behind a mask of suffering; and finally, I am tempted to say, a terminal holding off in perpetuity of a recognition of loss. For the deepest secret of the dead mother is that she never dies. No one ever has to die. Some secrets are too tempting to resist. A simple trade is sufficient: 'give your life over to me now and we will always remain together'.

The problem (that is, the symptom) only arises when one party wants out of the deal. The problem in the analysis of the dead mother complex is that another irresistible bargain is forged once we listen in on its secrets. A new covenant is inevitably whispered in the patient's ear, and we find ourselves offering the analysis as the latest version of an old alliance, as a new dead mother. For who really dares to awaken the dead from their sleep?

Bits and pieces

I want to change direction here, and focus on just a piece of an image. Nina had an occasional symptom, one of those symptoms that seem to arise in a session like an interesting piece of gossip, or an aside about the news, recognised as intriguing, but not really seen as central to matters at hand. The symptom consisted of a belief, a conviction really, that something disgusting was on her mouth. She would become preoccupied with this repulsive feeling, and would go to some lengths (a special towel, cool water, particular ways of cleaning) in the hope that she could wipe the feeling away. As I noted, Nina seemed subtly uninterested in this bit of her life, and it took a while before she paid much attention to it. When she did, several things became apparent. The disgusting mouth feeling arose under particular circumstances. She would have a period of feeling better, released and relieved. Then there would be the gnawing sense that something was coming undone. That she was no longer safe. Other thoughts would start to preoccupy her (health concerns or the image of her mother falling) but at the periphery of these worries, less a thought or an image than a tropism, there was the fear that she would *become* disgusting.

I have previously (Sekoff, 1994) described an 'abject triad', where fear, fascination, and bodily horror seize hold of the subject. Borrowing from Julia Kristeva's theorisation of abjection (Kristeva, 1982), I tried to chart a domain where the excreta of psychical life mark a kind of textured self, that is, where sensuous, but often repellent, textures of bodily experience are drawn upon to establish the boundaries and limits of psychic space. Perhaps another clinical story will help to explain this idea and its connection to the dead mother complex.

Helen B. arrived at her college film class to discover the students huddled around the one working monitor. She found a seat and settled in to watch the day's showing, *Chinatown*. Squeezing by her, a harried man, big and burly, wrestled himself into the next chair. She felt his presence with growing discomfort. He seemed to be crowding her out, sucking out the air. The room began to feel hot and the film appeared fuzzy. Suddenly, in panic, she leapt up and rushed down the aisle. As she stumbled over her unwelcome neighbour, her dangling purse bashed him on the head as she fled. Breathlessly, Helen related this story, complaining that I must do something about her 'out-of-control anger'. That she had been angry was clear enough; the purse made that point. Yet I wondered if offering her anger for repair served to distract from other upsetting contents. I told her that I was struck most by the intrusion she experienced. She responded, 'I felt invaded ... it made me feel crazy.' Several associations followed: she felt grossed out during a class film depicting elderly couples having sex. A television talk show about women's ejaculation evoked a similar response. She added thoughts about her panic: 'The worst thing was that the guy was chewing gum'. After some hesitation, she continued: 'It reminded me of my dog. This is horrible ... of my dog licking his testicles.' Recently, she had found herself worried about houseguests leaving the fluids of their lovemaking on her sheets. And she found herself disgusted by the sounds of her lover in the bathroom.

Why these sudden preoccupations? Like Nina, she had a depressed mother to contend with; however, Helen's mother had been less merging than disappearing, purposely working a night shift, leaving the children to fend for themselves during her sleep-filled days. It was her father who had filled the role of the object who could not be left. Alcoholic, her father seemed to treat Helen as a valued whisky – that is, highly prized and indulged in often. She commented after her panic attack, that 'he treats me like a possession. Worse, like a girlfriend. I could think my own thoughts if I had any room to breathe.'[2] Against this backdrop, I took the eruption of anxiety as a sign of Helen's struggle to create a psychic 'room of her own', a room apart from the jarring movement of absent or suffocating others. Now, three years into our treatment, Helen was occupied with boundaries and their connection to bodily and sexual phantasies. It is intriguing that *Chinatown*'s story of corruption, power, and incest was the background to her panic attack. Helen was grappling with her own vision of corruption ('textured currents', actual and phantasised) which blocked her path forward. Disgust, fear, loathing (the abject) marked the passage towards this threshold.

It is my contention that the abject appears at the boundary of self and other, usually at the site of a transition in psychic functioning. Abjection may function as an anchor, a handle, or a bridge across crucial thresholds of experience. At other times, the abject marks a retreat or punctuates a failure to cross a threshold. When Nina stood too long outside the shadow of the dead mother, she lost a needed anchorage. The abject broke her fall. Helen also reached out beyond a deadening inner landscape, only to fear for her sanity. The abject represented both a threat to her mental space, and a desperate means to staunch the flow of a rapidly shifting psychic field.

André Green holds out Winnicott's essay on 'The use of an object and relating through identifications' as a model for clinical approaches to the dead mother. In this paper, Winnicott leaves an intriguing footnote: 'the next task for a worker in the field of transitional phenomena is to restate the problem in terms of disposal' (Winnicott, 1968, p. 91). Crossing the threshold of transitional space entails leaving behind a waste product: a residue, a detritus, a shed skin. Perhaps the abject is precisely this residue: a disposal of psychic excreta, laden with the aggression and negativity that fuelled the cycle of destruction vital to transition and growth. Winnicott famously proposed that all authentic object relating depends upon an unconscious and continuous backcloth of destruction that releases the object from the subject's omnipotent control. Along these lines, perhaps the abject arises from the failure to tolerate the destruction inherent in object relating. The dead mother will not die, and only disgust and horror are left to mark the open grave.

Thinking back to Nina and Helen, might we now understand their bodily horrors as waste products of a transitional phase? The elements of object use appear to have been assembling – in their treatments each had begun to risk an aggression, a separateness, a bit of ruthlessness. Even so, each began to fall back under the inner conviction that their objects could not bear their destruction. Where the object was, the abject shall be. Indeed, patients in the orbit of the dead mother are extraordinarily sensitive to changes of state, to any signs of fluidity or flux. For example, if Nina got out of bed too quickly, felt a change in room temperature, had a sleep routine disrupted, sensed a food out of place in the kitchen, or faced the heightened in-between feeling of a trip, she was thrown into spasms of fear. Contingency was terrifying, indeterminacy the enemy.

In a series of studies, Ernst Hartmann has described 'boundary regulation' as a central property of all psychic functioning. His work focuses on variations in the 'thinness' and 'thickness' of psychic boundaries, delineating boundaries drawn intra-subjectively (between inside and outside), as well as intra-psychically (the borderlands between psychical states, between self and object representations) (Hartmann, 1991).

The intra-subjective boundaries of a psyche dominated by the dead mother complex appear quite thin – porous and permeable. On the one hand, this gives an attentive, loving, sympathetic quality to their interactions. On the other hand, they are left quite vulnerable to suggestion, intrusion, and impingement. Nina was thrown by the slightest hints of disapproval, conflict, or demand. Highly suggestible, she needed to be careful about what she read or overheard. A loving friend, she could be bruised easily, and turned her hurt quite harshly and fully upon her self. At the same time, the internal boundaries of the dead mother complex are quite thick, impermeable, fixed. Contradictory or multiple sets of thoughts and feelings are felt to be untenable. The flows and oscillations of mental/emotional life are anxiety provoking. There is a not-so-subtle attack on linking at work here, as if the organisation of the dead mother could not bear to contain the tidal currents of a psychical life that might carry the subject away from her rocky shores.

The abject, and indeed the dead mother complex itself, may be seen as special cases of the formation and regulation of psychic boundaries. While the 'textured self' is vital to these processes, the whole of psychical life, all of one's thoughts, phantasies, affects, and somatic registrations are brought to bear. What we find in the dead mother complex is an extraordinary vigilance, a relentless energy gathered around the proposition that no life is possible beyond the boundary of the dead mother's embrace. Peace of mind is a rare commodity in the dead mother complex. For in essence, the complex is a kind of death march within the mind, or more specifically, a kind of war of the mind against the self, against the soma, and against the affective resonances of the psyche. All spontaneous uprisings of the emotions, of the body, of phantasy, represent a threat to the regime of the dead mother. The mind is organised as an object whose function is to keep at bay, at all costs, any striving that might interrupt the vigilant watch of the subject over the vault of the 'dead objects'.

This mind-object (Corrigan and Gordon, 1995) is in essence a bulwark against movement, against changes of state. It is a keeper of boundaries, surveying the border between self and other, and guarding the oscillations and surprises of desire, emotion, and the drives. The mind-object serves to still any unfiltered activity, any unauthorised border crossings. More drastically, and often quite brutally, the functioning of the mind-object turns to what Green terms negative narcissism, a dissolution of the unity of the psyche, a movement that can only head one way: towards nothingness.

The dead and the undead

Death is often imagined as a kind of boundary or borderland. One crosses the River Styx to enter the realm of the dead. The moment of death in particular dizzies us with its dissolution of fundamental boundary lines – between the animate and the inanimate, between the present and the past, between presence and absence. Anthropologists call such blurred states 'liminal', where the usual rules of order, the acceptable modes of cultural transformation, are thrown into question. Though liminal states may evoke pleasure as well as fear, they compel rituals to compensate for their indeterminacy, and to tap into their aura of power. Last rites, last words, last wishes, death masks, funerary rites, mourning rules – all register the aura of death as it reverberates among the living. At the dawn of the photograph, another form of death, public executions, brought the dead regularly into view. By 1820, over 200 offences were capital crimes in England (Hay et al., 1975), and offenders as young as six years of age met their end at the gallows.[3;4] In this necrophilic atmosphere, public hangings were standard fare as a lesson for the assembled, as spectacle and sport, and also because the crowd demanded an accounting not only of the criminal, but of the Crown. The assembled wished to ensure proper procedures and a proper 'Christian' burial for one of their own. (Corpses had a nasty habit of turning up on the anatomist's table.) Sick children or ailing adults were often taken to the front of the crowd, in the belief that to gaze upon the condemned at the moment of death, or better, to touch their still warm hand the moment after, could effect a cure.

Such necromancy, that is, the attempt to harness the liminal power of death, may be central to the dead mother complex. Several patients recalled with crystal clarity a moment of death, or rather a moment like a thunderclap, when they felt filled with the possibility that their parent could die. This shattering awareness prompted feverish attempts to insure against the catastrophe: phantasies of outwitting death (time machines, medical cures, cryogenics), phobias about funerals or obituaries, and as we have seen, disavowal of the instruments that might bring about death: anger, separateness, conflict. Within the dead mother complex, the necromancer offers their own warm hand, held against the cold cheek of the fading other.

It seems no longer possible in this discussion to neglect a key question: why invoke the 'dead', what is 'dead' about the dead mother? After all, everything Green points to reminds us that this is a peculiarly lively corpse. Indeed, few of the living exercise such vital power. So is all this talk of 'the dead' mere hyperbole, a metaphor gone awry?

In his remarkable, 'Thoughts for the times on war and death', Freud quoted the proverb, 'To think about something as though it were death' (1915), that is to say, not to think about it at all. Psychoanalysis has a history of beckoning death into its reach, only to have it pushed away again. Death hardly sits with sex, or attachment, or the self at the centre of recent analytic discourse. Attempts to think again on the subject, such as Green's or Ogden's (this volume) description of deadness as a fundamental psychic entity, have drawn criticism for having too grim a vocabulary, when we have other, less exaggerated descriptions to put to work. Yet, can death be banished so easily? With the dawning of the modern era, death began to recede from the front parlour or the bedroom to the funeral home and the hospital suite. So, too, has death retreated from the lingua franca of psychoanalytic discourse, to be left to the occasional new age prophet, or self-help programme.

Thankfully, much of this denial of death stems from the reduction of death's presence among us, largely due to public health measures available to the fortunate of the West. The romantic cult of death in the Victorian era (tubercular heroines and doomed, angelic children) was less do to with the Victorians' superior moral fibre than the unavoidable presence of so many familiar deceased. If today we hark back to a closer linkage to death, we do so from the safety of approaching a relative stranger.[5]

Still, all those photographs of dead children were also nudged off the mantlepiece when death proved an inconvenient companion to the modern consumer spectacle. In the first decade of this century, the *Ladies' Home Journal* began a campaign to banish the word *parlour* from our vocabularies. 'Living Rooms' were to be a place of light and new appliances and any reminders of the death-ridden parlour were censored from the pages of the influential women's magazine. Perhaps we have encountered some psychoanalytic house-cleaning as well? No need to be too troubled by those figures of the *ancien régime*: sex, death, and the unconscious (Sekoff, 1977).

'But these neurotics', Freud wrote in the analysis of the Rat Man, 'need the help of the possibility of death chiefly in order that it may act as a solution of conflicts they have left unsolved' (Freud, 1909, p. 236). We all need to take full measure of death, if only to face the question, what is it to be alive? Freud suggests that we cannot hope to approach an answer, unless we are prepared to encounter transience, the fading and passing of ourselves and our objects.[6]

It is striking how often the thematic of death surfaces in Nina's story: gravestones, suicide, dead ears, dead friends. Death dances through her life, while liveliness is frozen, suspended. This is less an engagement with death (though the dead are clearly a familiar presence) than an entombment. In an odd way, all the thoughts of death keep its presence at bay, like conversations after a funeral, it is only when the talking stops that the loss is fully felt. Death surrounded Nina not only as an extension of loss, but because murder was in the air. Green returns us to Freud in his refusal to subsume murder within the term aggression. With Freud, he charts the killing field of the dead mother: a murderous envy that the dead mother holds for the living, and a killing rage that those held in her grasp carry within them. As any homicide detective could point out, there are a variety of motives for murder, but they all have the same aim: to eliminate an other who is in one's way.

Freud noted one murderous variant, again in the case of the Rat Man: 'In his imagination … he was constantly making away with people so as to show his heartfelt sympathy for their bereaved relatives' (Freud, 1909, p. 235). Green notes another, when he describes a desire to kill the object in 'order to find shelter in a mythic self-sufficiency' (1986c, p. 27). As we listen for the dead mother, we must hear the whispers of the adoring child: 'Die, leave me be, let me go.' Killing her softly, death becomes her.

So here we might finally say that dead mother is a misnomer, not for its exaggeration, but because 'dead' doesn't fully capture the power of this object. We find an object that is more accurately described as 'compressing' or 'entrapping' rather than lifeless. A centrifuge object whose gravity won't let anything escape. In another vocabulary it is bad rather than absent, whether re-introjecting projections of envy and hatred (Klein), or as a repository of unmet need (Fairbairn). Above all, to borrow an idea of Anne Alvarez, it is a useless object (Alvarez, 1997). That is, the dead mother fails in its role of providing a refuge of sufficient strength and flexibility to allow the subject to leave it behind. In sum, we find less a dead object, than an object that is deadening. In the cinema of horror, it is the zombie, the walking dead who seek out the living to add them to their deadened numbers. These 'undead' with their stiffened gait, decomposing flesh, and relentless gaze seem to need the living – as if envying the existence of those who still inhabit the light and walk freely. As one adolescent described the zombie he drew, 'He's lonely for others.' Yet it is not so much life the undead pursue than a respite from their half dead/half alive torture. Death is not the enemy; the horror is to be suspended between life and death.

This is the fate of the dead and deadening object relations of the dead mother complex: to be suspended between the living and the dead. John Steiner (1993) has written of a half-dead state where both object and self are tormented, but not allowed to die. This state is a psychic retreat from the full measure of guilt and loss that separation from objects entails. In such a state, it is the agency of the subject (an agency brimming with desire, aggression, sex, murder, sufficiency, separateness) that remains suspended. Psychic retreat (or in Jean Wolff Bernstein's felicitous phrase, psychic exile) is an attempt to assuage the angry gods by playing dead (Wolf-Bernstein, 1996).

How did Nina play dead? In part, by imagining her own death by various means – illness, poisoning, accidents, hanging up the phone. In part, by turning her back on the living when stepping forward too noisily might awaken the undead. In part, by becoming her maternal imago: matching pain for pain, worry for worry. Most of all, by turning her desire into a cemetery of refusals, suspending the most basic claim of the living upon the dead: to be left in peace.

Burying the dead

And what of the necromancy of the psychoanalytic encounter? Are we conjuring up the dead, or finding stakes to put through the hearts of the wandering zombies? It is late in the day and we must leave for another time a fuller encounter with Green's enriching ideas. Still, to linger over the question a moment longer: if we keep in mind that it is not death *per se* that we are contending with, but stasis – the freezing of movement across psychic pathways – then we are not left to peddle the necromancer's art. We can put aside their potions and incantations and instead seek to discover the art of living in the liminal. Indeed, Green utilises Winnicott's epistemology to anchor such a clinical approach. It is paradox, above all, that Winnicott hopes to tolerate in himself and within his patients. (Even if Green takes Winnicott to task for undervaluing the paradox of sex.) In Winnicott's œuvre of the 'in-between', we come to see the essential structuring effects of a potential space wherein the flow of psychic life may be engaged.

In many ways, Nina and Helen were still perched on the comforting gravestones of their childhood, and it was no small task to interest them in what lay beyond the cemetery walls, for they already knew what awaited: the terrible loss of a moment of aliveness, of a place where they were held within their mother's gaze. To coax the subject beyond their funeral vault demands a psychoanalysis of 'paradoxical absence'. That is to say, the therapeutic task is to raise the possibility of constituting absence, in place of an adherence to undeadness. Yet, this absence must re-present an opening out, up, or into a potential presence. In Green's language, the some-thing of absence must take the space of the no-thing that the dead mother 'unpresents'.[7]

This is all a bit abstract. Even Green's call for a *discours vivant*, a language alive with affect, leaves us waiting for more concrete guidance – for who among us feels that they approach their patients with a deadened voice?

I am reminded of another patient, who could be an analytic cousin of the patients we have met. Bright, creative, loving, yet captured in his soul by a pledge to an inner other, Mark also suffered the pains of trading a separate life for the comforts of the dead mother. In one session, he told me of a phone call to a friend who was suffering horrible panic attacks, a symptom he himself shared. In their conversation, Mark commented that, 'you seem to be afraid of moving forward, as if any movement from you is like the creation of dead bodies'. This interpretation was not simply a case of borrowing the words of the analysis to pass on uninvited to others (something most of us have been guilty of with our own patients). The 'creation of dead bodies' was a newly felt thought for Mark. It is a truism that our surest, most meaningful interpretations are also in some measure spoken to ourselves. Mark's words did such double duty. A doubling in another sense also, for his words invited his friend to think of the dualities of her dilemma: separation as aggression, movement as murder, panic as stasis.

To 'feel the thought' is a complex act, constituted not only through the linking of emotion with cognition, but also when we are able to embody a lived object relationship that links self and other, affect and object, past and present. Green helps us to see that all 'felt thoughts' are both shadow and light, that is, the presence of our psychic experience rests on a penumbra of absence. In the lived experience of the analytic relationship, 'felt thoughts' and 'thought feelings' are constructed, or better, incubated both between and within each member of the analytic couple. At the boundary of self and other we risk encountering each other's shadow and light (that is, we take up the chance of both mutuality and negation, of reciprocity as well as conflict). It is in this risk that the analytic object may potentially be discovered.

One last clinical story. For two weeks running, Linda M. had awakened in abject terror from the same dream. Not only had she dreamt the identical dream each night, but she had awakened at precisely the same time, 3:23 a.m. In the dream, she awakens in her bedroom to an uneasy feeling that she is not alone. As she looks up and out of her window, she makes out bodies, faces, staring in at her through the pane. With a shudder, she recognises the gathering: they are dead relatives, each and every one, and they are beckoning to her, urging her through their gazes to come join them. Her associations to the dreams were quite sparse; that is, she was left after the dream as she felt inside the dreams: quite speechless, caught by the look of her lost loved ones.

We knew the context for the dreams: Linda had lived through a hurricane, huddled in her windswept bedroom and terrified that she would join the dearly departed. The dreams were ripe with the trauma of the event, and we were at an anniversary. We wondered together about the lingering sense of terror and helplessness, but also of a wish to cross over, to find relief in the ghostly embrace of her missed and yearning dead. Beyond the content of the dreams, their timing and persistence were most striking. Linda was focused on the pain/pane of the dream and showed a lack of curiosity about the dreaming itself. This seemed an absence worth pursuing. I asked her why she appeared so unmoved by the precision of the awakening, though she had made note of its unyielding rhythm. She agreed this was curious, but again felt dried up in her thoughts.

The dream as an object of the treatment had made a dramatic appearance, only to run aground on this (dry) shoal. What course to pursue? The temptation was to engage in what might be called the 'detective trope' of analysis, a hot pursuit of hidden meanings. Another course would be to avoid such enticements and return to the drying up as our point of interest. A third tactic, somewhere between the two, emerged – perhaps more along the lines of our trope of 'incubation'. I told her that my own association, relevant or not, was to another anniversary, which had appeared in our work years ago, only to 'dry up' quickly. She had spoken once or twice about a broken engagement to a young man whom she had loved very much.

Linda thought it odd that I should remember this now. She didn't see the connection, although, come to think of it, she had had a thought about this failed romance, for the first time in years, just the other day. She painfully remembered his cruelty to her. He broke off their relationship the night of their first sexual encounter. Venomously, he told her that she disgusted him, that he thought her a whore (though she was a virgin), and that he wanted no more of her. They were to have been married on March 23rd. Three, Two, Three. We both seemed less interested at that point in deciding if this numeric magic reflected the uncanny calculations of the unconscious, or an unconscious calculation that accommodated the numbers to meet my association. What was most important was that a *discours vivant* had emerged. She went on to recount the pain of that time, the deep questioning of her feelings, perceptions, and sexuality. These doubts were still with her; she now connected her misgivings to an earlier set of doubts: her parents had not approved of her romance, indeed, of any activity that took her too far from home. She wondered how the dream might be connected to a time when she had stepped forward, only to be thrown back bruised and chastened.

Another sequence of associations followed. She recalled her phobia for rhythmic noises; since childhood she would grow anxious at repetitive sounds. The dream of the dead relatives had a kind of rhythm to it: the undead seemed to look on in unison, and even, she now recalled, stood tapping on the window. We had crossed this terrain previously, encountering phantasies about the rhythms of her parents' bedroom, which she had shared as a child in latency. I now recalled another rhythm: her mother sometimes expressed her depressed mood by slowly and solidly knocking her own head against the wall. Linda had been terrified at the sight of her mother's behaviour. She was helpless to stop it, no matter what tearful, begging pleas she made. At night, she would sneak into her parent's bedroom to check if her mother was still breathing. She also made an inner pledge: to act so much nicer, to be so much better, anything, just so the terrible banging would stop. After this session's dream-work, the dream cycle continued, but with something new put into motion. The gathered relatives seemed clearer, their faces less ghost-like, more lively. And someone else came into the dream: her dead father, with a hunting rifle in hand, asking her to join him in a chase. The paternal appearance reminds us of another absence in our encounter with the dead mother, a missing third figure, who might offer some inducement away from the world of the dead, but who seems to arrive always too late in the day.

It is indeed late in the day. We must leave to others a fuller encounter with Green's enriching idea. I am aware of what has gone wanting in this exposition, as much as what has been addressed. In addition to the paternal dynamics which have been slighted, we have barely touched the erotic play (and at times the erotic misery) that greet the analytic couple who find their way into the sanctum of the dead mother.

Thinking back on the photographs of the dead children, we may reflect on the fundamental pathos of trying to hold within the mind's eye what the world has taken away. Nina and Helen had each faced such pathos: a world of depressed intensities, both absent and demanding. Each in her own way sought to turn back the night as the dark sun of their mother's face closed the world tight around them (Kristeva, 1987). And each in her own way had to find her own gaze, her own way of looking back at the maternal image that threatened to hold her, just as frozen, just as loved, and just as lost as those dead children.

Hans Loewald once described psychoanalysis as turning ghosts into ancestors. André Green has given us a psychoanalysis of absence that imagines the possibility of both ghosts and ancestors coming to rest in a lively peace.

Notes

1   'Sublime' also evokes 'sublimation', and Green speaks of the remarkable capacity for associative and artistic creation emanating out of the struggle with negativity. Yet these 'precocious idealized sublimations' fail to address the wound at the core of the patient. A lesser-known definition of sublime speaks to this wound. Sublime: 'to cause to pass directly from the solid to the vapor state' (Merriam-Webster, 1989).

2   To make things worse, the psychiatrist the family consulted when Helen was 16 managed to sleep with her mother, chase after Helen with marriage proposals, and later get himself arrested for selling drugs.

3   The number of capital offences – almost all for property crimes – rose from about 20 in 1600 to over 200. However, the rate of executions remained relatively

stable – the use of pardons and emigration being widespread. Hanging days were big social events and many social upheavals accompanied them, including the Tyburn Riot of 1749, when the crowd rose up against the surgeons they saw as stealing the bodies of the condemned (see Hay *et al.*, 1975).

4   Many funerary rites recognise the intensities of somato-psychic life that are evoked as the dead begin their journey across the boundary that had previously delimited life from death. When death comes to the Cashinau of the Peruvian Amazon, the community gathers round the now still body. Wails of distress rise up from the assembled and the woeful cries unleash a stream of secretions – tears, mucus, and saliva spewing forth from eyes, nose and mouth. The mourners gather up the products of their sorrow and wrap the dead body in the viscous fluids of the tribe. A proper death, a good death, is sealed by this glistening body tomb (Kenssinger, 1973).

5   Though for some communities and patients (children of the inner city, gay men) death looms all too close.

6   I am indebted to Serge Leclaire's discussion of Freud's thoughts on death and death-work in the essay, 'Jerome, or death in the life of the obsessional' (1980).

7   Rachael Peltz (1996; 1998) has taken up the dialectic of presence and absence in a number of contexts. She explores this thematic as it relates to the construction of self and subjectivity; the constitution of the psychoanalytic couple; and pertinently, to the dead mother complex itself. Also, among contributors to the present volume, previous work of Michael Parsons (1996) and Gregorio Kohon (1986) takes up this dialectic as well.

References

Alvarez, A.(1997) Presentation to the Child Analytic Program of the San Francisco Psychoanalytic Institute. February 1997.

Anzieu, D. (ed.) (1990) *Psychic Envelopes*. London: Karnac Books.

Barthes, R. (1981) *Camera Lucida*. New York: Hill and Wang.

Bion, W.(1959) Attacks on linking. *International Journal of Psycho-analysis* 40: 308–15.

Corrigan, E. and Gordon, P. E. (1995) *The Mind Object*. Northvale, NJ: Jason Aronson.

Freud, S. (1909) Notes upon a case of obsessional neurosis. *S.E.* 10.

—— (1911) *Totem and Taboo*. *S.E.* 13.

—— (1915) Thoughts for the times on war and death. *S.E.* 14.

—— (1917) Mourning and melancholia. *S.E.* 14.

Goldberg, P. (1995) 'Successful' dissociation, pseudo vitality, and inauthentic use of the senses. *Psychoanalytic Dialogues* 5(3):493–510.

Green, A. (1983) The dead mother. In *On Private Madness*. Madison, CT: International Universities Press.

—— (1986a) The analyst, symbolization and absence in the analytical setting. In *On Private Madness*. Madison, CT: International Universities Press.

—— (1986b) Potential space in psychoanalysis. In *On Private Madness*. Madison, CT: International Universities Press.

—— (1986c) Psychoanalysis and ordinary modes of thought. In *On Private Madness*. Madison, CT: International Universities Press.

Hartmann, E. (1991) *Boundaries in the Mind*. New York: Basic Books.

Hay, D. *et al.* (1975) *Albion's Fatal Tree*. New York: Pantheon.

Kenssinger, K. (1973) Personal communication.

Kohon, G. (1986) Countertransference: An independent view. In G. Kohon (ed.) *The British School of Psychoanalysis: The Independent Tradition*. New Haven: Yale University Press.

Kristeva, J. (1982) *Powers of Horror*. New York: Colombia University Press.

—— (1987) *Black Sun: Depression and Melancholia*. New York: University Press.

Leclaire, S. (1980) Jerome, or death in the life of the obsessional. In S. Schneiderman *Returning to Freud*. New Haven: Yale University Press.

New Merriam-Webster Dictionary (1989) Springfield, MA; Merriam-Webster Publishers.

Ogden, T. (1997) Analysing forms of aliveness and deadness of the transference–countertransference (in this current volume).

Parsons, M. (1996) Recent work by André Green. *International Journal of Psycho-Analysis* 77: 399–406.

Peltz, R, (1990) Mr. Nobody: The dead mother complex and the psychogenesis of character and sexual identity problems. (Presentation to the annual spring meeting of the Division of psychoanalysis of the American Psychological Association. Boston, 1994.) Unpublished.

—— (1998) The dialectic of presence and absence: Impasses and the retrieval of meaning states. *Psychoanalytic Dialogues*, May-June, Vol. 8 (3), pp. 385–409.

Sekoff, J. (1977) Down they forgot, as up they grew: The organizations of children's play in industrializing America. Unpublished thesis. Amherst: Hampshire College.

—— (1994) Blue Velvet: The surface of suffering. *Free Associations* 4(3): 31:421–46.

Steiner, J. (1993) *Psychic Retreats*. London: Routledge.

Sontag, S. (1977) *On Photography*. New York: Dell Publishing.

Upton, B. (1976) *Photography*. Boston: Little Brown.

Warner, M. (1995) Stealing souls and catching shadows. *TATE: The Art Magazine*, 6 Summer, pp. 40–7.

Winnicott, D. W. (1963) Fear of breakdown. *International Review of Psycho-Analysis*, 1, pp. 103–7, 1974.

Winnicott, D. W. (1971) The use of an object and relating through identifications. In *Playing and Reality*. London: Tavistock.

—— (1974) Fear of breakdown. *International Review of Psycho-Analysis* 1: 103–7. Also in G. Kohon (ed.). *The British School of Psychoanalysis: The Independent Tradition*. New Haven: Yale University Press, 1986.

Wolff Bernstein, J. (1996) Discussion of John Steiner's 'Revenge, retreat and resentment'. Psychoanalytic Institute of Northern California. November 1996. Unpublished manuscript.

6

ANALYSING FORMS OF ALIVENESS AND DEADNESS OF THE TRANSFERENCE– COUNTERTRANSFERENCE

Thomas H. Ogden

The Other Tiger

We'll hunt for a third tiger now, but like
The others this one too will be a form
Of what I dream, a structure of words, and not
The flesh and bone tiger that beyond all myths
Paces the earth. I know these things quite well,
Yet nonetheless some force keeps driving me
In this vague, unreasonable, and ancient quest,
And I go on pursuing through the hours
Another tiger, the beast not found in verse.

(J. L. Borges, 1960)

I have become increasingly aware over the past several years that the sense of aliveness and deadness of the transference–countertransference is, for me, perhaps the single most important measure of the moment-to-moment status of the analytic process. In the course of four clinical discussions, I shall explore the idea that an essential element of analytic technique involves the analyst's making use of his experience in the countertransference to address specific expressive and defensive roles of the sense of aliveness and deadness of the analysis as well as the particular function of these qualities of experience in the landscape of the patient's internal object world and object relationships. From this perspective, the problems of central concern to analyst and analysand tend to focus increasingly on such questions as: when was the last time the analysis felt alive to both participants?; is there a disguised vitality that cannot be acknowledged by analyst and/or analysand for fear of the consequences of its recognition?; what sorts of substitute formations might be masking the lifelessness of the analysis, e.g. manic excitement, perverse pleasure, hysterical acting-in and acting out, as if constructions, parasitic dependence on the inner life of the analyst, and so on?

The ideas that I shall present are based in large part on Winnicott's (1971) conception of the 'place where we live' (a third area of experiencing between reality and fantasy (1951)) and the problems involved in generating such a 'place' (intersubjective state of mind) in the analysis. I am also drawing heavily upon Bion's (1959) notion that the analyst/mother keeps alive, and in a sense brings to life, the analysand's/infant's projected aspects of self through the successful containment of projective identifications. Symington's (1983) and Coltart's (1986) discussions of the analyst's freedom to think, represent important applications to analytic technique of the work of Bion and Winnicott. Green (1983) has made a pivotal contribution to the analytic understanding of the experience of deadness as an early internalisation of the unconscious state of the depressed mother.

A great deal has been written in recent years about the importance of the analyst's 'realness', i.e. his/her capacity for spontaneity and freedom to respond to the analysand from his/her own experience in the analytic situation in a way that is not strangulated by stilted caricatures of analytic neutrality (see for example, Bollas, 1987; Casement, 1985; Meares, 1993; Mitchell, 1993; Stewart, 1977). As will be clinically illustrated, my own technique rarely includes discussing the countertransference with the patient directly. Instead, the countertransference[1] is implicitly presented in the way I conduct myself as an analyst, for example, in the management of the analytic frame, the tone, wording and content of interpretations and other interventions, in the premium that is placed on symbolisation as opposed to tension-dissipating action, and so on.

I shall attempt to develop several ideas having to do with technical problems involved in recognising, symbolising and interpreting the sense of aliveness and deadness of the analytic experience. I believe that every form of psychopathology represents a specific type of limitation of the individual's capacity to be fully alive as a human being. The goal of analysis from this point of view is larger than that of the resolution of unconscious intrapsychic conflict, the diminution of symptomatology, the enhancement of reflective subjectivity and self-understanding, and the increase of sense of personal agency. Although one's sense of being alive is intimately intertwined with each of the above-mentioned capacities, I believe that the experience of aliveness is a quality that is superordinate to these capacities and must be considered as an aspect of the analytic experience *in its own terms*.

The focus of this chapter is clinical. My effort will not be to define psychological aliveness and deadness or even to attempt to describe how we determine whether, or to what extent, a given experience has the quality of aliveness or of deadness. It is not that these questions are unimportant. Rather, the best way I have of addressing these questions is to discuss clinical situations that I believe centrally involve these qualities of experience and to hope that the descriptions themselves convey something of a sense of the ways in which aliveness and deadness are consciously and unconsciously experienced by analyst and analysand. In the four clinical discussions of forms of psychological aliveness and deadness that follow, particular attention is paid to the ways in which countertransference experience is utilised in the process of creating analytic meaning, i.e. in the process of recognising, symbolising, understanding and interpreting the leading transference–countertransference anxiety.

I

In the first clinical discussion, I will present fragments of an analysis in which the patient's sense of deadness could not initially be symbolised and instead was enacted (entombed) in the lifelessness of the analytic experience itself. The focus of this discussion will be on the use of the countertransference to generate verbal symbols that are eventually offered to the patient in the form of interpretations.

Ms N., a highly successful civic leader, began analysis because she felt intense, but diffuse anxiety and believed that something was seriously wrong in her life, but did not know what it was. In the initial meetings the patient did not seem to consciously experience feelings of emptiness, futility or stagnation. She said that she felt at a loss for words, which was something that was highly uncharacteristic of her.

The first year and a half of analysis in many ways had the appearance of a satisfactory beginning. The patient was able to see more clearly the specific ways in which she kept people (including me) at a great psychological distance. There was also some decrease in anxiety which was reflected in the patient's increasingly less rigid body posture on the couch. (For almost a year, Ms N. had lain completely still on the couch with her hands folded on her stomach. At the end of the meeting, the patient would bolt from the couch and briskly leave the room without looking at me.) The language the patient used was initially equally stiff and often sounded textbookish. Her speech pattern became somewhat more natural in the course of the initial year of work. However, the patient throughout this period had profound doubts about whether the analysis was of 'any real value' to her. Ms N. felt that she was developing no greater understanding of either the source of her anxiety or of her sense that things were not right in her life.

In the course of the first half of the second year of work, I gradually developed an awareness of the way in which the patient would fill the hours with apparently introspective talk that did not seem to develop into elements from which further understanding or interpretation could be generated. A pattern developed in the hours in which Ms N. would describe events in her life in minute detail. It was not at all clear what the point of the lengthy descriptions was. At times, I would say to the patient that I thought that she must be very anxious that I would learn too much about her if she helped me to understand the significance of what she had just said.

I found that I experienced increasingly less curiosity about the patient, which absence had quite a disturbing effect on me. It felt equivalent to losing the use of my mind. I experienced a form of claustrophobia during the hours and on occasion defended against this anxiety by obsessionally counting the minutes until the hour would be over. At other times, I fantasised ending the hour prematurely by telling the patient that I was ill and needed to end the session. I would sometimes 'pass the time' by counting the beats per minute of my radial pulse. I was initially unaware that there was anything odd about my taking my pulse despite the fact that this is a practice that has never occurred with any other patient. As the thoughts, feelings, and sensations associated with this activity were occurring, they did not feel like 'analytic data'. Instead, I experienced them as an almost invisible, private background experience.

During the period of weeks that followed, I gradually became more able to treat the taking of my pulse, as well as the associated feelings and sensations, as 'analytic objects' (Bion, 1962; Green, 1975; Ogden, 1994a, d), i.e. as a reflection of an unconscious construction being generated by the patient and myself, or more accurately being generated by the 'intersubjective analytic third'. I have discussed my conception of the 'intersubjective analytic third' (or 'the analytic third') in a recent series of publications (Ogden, 1992a, b, 1994a, b, c, d). To briefly summarise the ideas presented in those publications, the intersubjective analytic third is understood as a third subject created by the unconscious interplay of analyst and analysand; at the same time, the analyst and analysand qua analyst and analysand are generated in the act of creating the analytic third. (There is no analyst, no analysand, no analysis, aside from the process through which the analytic third is generated.)

The new subjectivity (the analytic third) stands in dialectical tension with the individual subjectivities of analyst and analysand. The intersubjective analytic third is not conceived of as a static entity; rather, it is understood as an evolving experience that is continually in a state of flux as the intersubjectivity of the analytic process is transformed by the understandings generated by the analytic pair.

The analytic third is experienced through the individual personality systems of analyst and analysand and is therefore not an identical experience for each. The creation of the analytic third reflects the asymmetry of the analytic situation in that it is created in the context of the analytic setting, which is structured by the relationship of roles of analyst and analysand. The unconscious experience of the analysand is privileged in the analytic relationship: it is the experience of the analysand (past and present) that is taken by the analyst and analysand as the principal (although not exclusive) subject of the analytic dialogue.

I began to be able to link the experience of holding my own wrist (in the act of taking my pulse) with what I now suspected to be a need to literally feel human warmth in an effort to reassure myself that I was alive and healthy. This realisation brought with it a profound shift in my understanding of a great many aspects of my experience with Ms N. I felt moved by the patient's tenacity in telling me seemingly pointless stories for more than 18 months. It occurred to me that these stories had been offered with the unconscious hope that I might find (or create) a point to the stories, thereby creating a point (a feeling of coherence, direction, value and authenticity) for the patient's life. I had previously been conscious of my own fantasy of feigning illness in order to escape the stagnant deadness of the sessions, but I had not understood that this 'excuse' reflected an unconscious fantasy that I was being made ill by prolonged exposure to the lifelessness of the analysis. It was through this and similar lines of thought and feeling (associated with my own experience in the analytic third) that I began to develop a sense of the meaning of the patient's diffuse anxiety and her sense that she was caught in something awful that she could not identify.

I said to Ms N. that I thought I understood better now some of the reasons for her telling me in great detail about events in her life in a way that made why she was telling the story confusing to both of us. I said that I felt that she had given up on being able to create a life for herself. Instead, she was giving me the forms with which she had filled her time in hopes that I could create a life for her from these pieces. The patient responded by describing the way in which her life at work and at home consisted almost entirely of organising other people's activities while never actually making anything herself. It now seemed to her that she used other people's lives and the things that they made (the lives of her employees, her husband, her au pair, and her two children) as a substitute for her own ability to create something that felt like a life of her own.

Later in the session, she said that she had for a long time imagined that a paperweight on a table next to my chair had been a gift from a patient. She said that she had never told me that she had even noticed the object, but that she had for a long time wished that she had given it to me. It was not until that moment that she realised that she had not imagined giving me a gift of her own, and instead had wished that she had given me *that gift*. She could not envision herself as a person who could select, and in that sense create, a gift for me, so she imagined being someone else, the person who had given me the gift. I thought, but did not interpret at this juncture, that underlying this thought was the fantasy that it would never be possible for her to create a life of her own so the only alternative available to her was that of stealing the life of another person. It seemed important that I not usurp the patient's opportunity to create life in the analysis (create interpretations) that she was now just beginning to be able to do.

Several months later, Ms N. presented a dream in which she was in a cabinet in a kitchen that was not her own kitchen. It was as if she had been 'poured into the cabinet' and had become a rectangular cube the shape of the inside of the wooden box. The dream was presented in conjunction with the patient's telling me about a friend who lived with continual psychological pain in connection with the death of her 5-year old daughter. The friend's child had been killed before the patient began analysis in an accident that had resulted from the negligence of a baby-sitter.

After telling me the dream, Ms N. fell silent. This silence stood in marked contrast to the way in which she had in the past obscured feeling with verbiage. After a few minutes, I said to Ms N. that I thought that she was describing to me her sense that she lacked a shape of her own. I went on to say that her friend's pain, however terrible, was a human feeling that I thought the patient feared she was incapable of experiencing. I told her that although she had never said so directly, I felt that she was afraid that she might never be able to feel anything, even the pain that others might feel about the death of their child.

In a voice so faint that I could barely hear her, Ms N. said that this had for a long time been a fear of hers about which she felt enormous shame. She had stayed awake many nights worrying that she would be unable to grieve if one of her own children were to die and that this felt to her to be the most odious failure of which any mother could be guilty. She said that she felt that she had not been able to love and be with her children in the way that she wished she could have been. In fact, she now knew that she had neglected them quite badly and that they had suffered greatly for it. The patient again fell silent for the remaining few minutes of the hour.

To summarise, I view the portion of the analysis just discussed as representing the beginnings of a process in which the patient's experience of deadness (both in her imagined inability to grieve and in her identification with her friend's dead child) was being transformed from an unthinkable thing-in-itself (a fact experienced by both the patient and myself as a non-verbally symbolised sense of deadness of the analysis) into a living, verbally symbolised experience of the patient's (and my own) deadness in the analysis. An intersubjective analytic space had begun to be generated in which the deadness could be felt, viewed, experienced and spoken about by the two of us. Deadness had become a feeling as opposed to a fact.

II

In this second clinical discussion, I shall describe an analytic encounter which illustrates technical challenges arising in conjunction with a patient's unconscious insistence that the analyst serve as the repository for his psychic life and hope.

Mr D., in the initial interview, informed me that he had been in analysis six times and each time 'had been terminated' by the analyst. The most recent unilateral termination had occurred three months prior to Mr D.'s first meeting with me.

The patient carried himself and spoke in a way that conveyed a sense of arrogance, aloofness and self-importance; at the same time, this deportment had a brittleness to it that made it readily apparent that the patient's superior tone of voice and demeanour thinly disguised feelings of fear, worthlessness and desperation.

Mr D. told me that if he were to continue past our initial meeting, I must understand that he would never be the one who spoke first in any session. He explained that if I were to attempt to 'wait him out,' the session would be spent in complete silence. He had wasted his time and money in that way too many times in the past and hoped that I would not repeat that approach with him. He added that it would also be a waste of time for me to ask him about the 'fears and anxieties' underlying his inability to begin the session: 'After all, my answering questions of that sort would be tantamount to my beginning the hour – you know that as well as I do.'

Mr D.'s presentation of himself intrigued me and stirred feelings of com-petitiveness in me. He had thrown down the gauntlet and I would prove myself to be more adept and agile than the previous six analysts. In the initial interview I was also aware that I was unconsciously being invited to take the role of a suitor and that there was a fantasised homosexual sadomasochistic scene that was already beginning to take shape in the transference–countertransference. At the same time, I recognised that the fantasy of entering into a competitive game protected me from fully feeling the deadly seriousness of the intense contempt and hatred that I was encountering. In addition, the narcissistic/competitive fantasy protected me from feelings of being trapped in the web that Mr D. was already beginning to spin with his imperiously controlling instructions regarding the way in which the analysis was to be conducted. I imagined that long years of isolation awaited both of us if we were to undertake analysis together.

I said to Mr D. that I thought he imagined that analysis with me would involve one or both of us brutalising the other until the one being brutalised could no longer bear it. I also said that I had no interest in brutalising him, being brutalised by him or participating in his brutalisation of himself. This comment was not meant as a reassurance, but as a statement about my conception of the analytic framework within which I was willing to work. I agreed to be the first to speak in each hour, but said that I would do so only when I thought I had something to say. I added that it might sometimes take me a good deal of time to be able to put my experience into words for myself and for him at the beginning of the session, but my silence would not be intended as an attempt to 'wait him out'.

Mr D. sat quietly and seemed to relax a bit as I spoke. I was somewhat encouraged by the fact that I felt that I had been able to say something to him that did not involve a sadistic attack on Mr D. nor a compromise of either of us. Neither did it seem to me to involve a form of manic excitement and denial related to the fantasy of a competitive game.

At the outset of each of the meetings with Mr D., I attempted to find words to convey what it felt like being with him in that particular moment. I (silently) hypothesised that both the fantasies and feelings about brutalisation and the fantasies reflecting manic excitement (competition) in the transference–countertransference represented forms of defence against the experience of inner deadness, which deadness was symbolised by Mr D.'s feeling that he had nothing in him with which to begin the hours (to begin his story). I would have to be the one to bring life to the analysis (to create history) each time we met. Almost always as I began the hour, I had the conscious fantasy that I was giving the patient and the analysis mouth-to-mouth resuscitation. I chose not to tell Mr D. about this fantasy directly in order not to demean him or to prematurely address the homosexual aspects of the transference–countertransference.

At times, what I said to Mr D. to begin the hour felt rote and hackneyed and I laboured to get beyond what felt like pre-fabricated analytic cliché in order not to dump further lifelessness into him and into the analysis. In one of these meetings very early on in the analysis I told Mr D. that I had found myself imagining attempting to lure him into trusting me. I said that I knew that this would not only be futile, but would also be destructive since anything 'won' by me in this way would be experienced by both of us as a form of theft that would alienate us from one another even further than we already were. After several minutes of silence, Mr D. described his continual vigilance in combating theft: his use of burglar alarms at his home, anti-theft devices in his car, a safe at his office, and so on. This was spoken in a way that gave no acknowledgement that it represented a response to what I had just said. Despite the patient's offering information of this sort, the feeling in the hour was that of an extremely tense stand-off which threatened to break apart at any moment. It felt as if there were nothing human holding the fabric of the analysis together.

In a session that occurred in the sixth month of the analysis, I thought for a moment that I saw tears brimming in Mr D.'s eyes, but when I looked more closely I could not tell if my perception had been accurate. (Mr D. was at that point refusing to use the couch and so we were meeting face to face.) I told Mr D. what had just occurred and said that whether or not there had been tears in his eyes, I felt that what had happened reflected the sadness of the situation that he and I were in. (I remembered Mr D.'s telling me some months earlier that he had been grateful to his previous analyst for her honesty in telling him that she could not be of help to him instead of mindlessly persisting in an analysis that she felt could not progress. That thought reminded me of a 'living will' that had recently been sent to me by a member of my family in which doctors were in effect instructed not to create an empty illusion of life after genuine life had already been lost.)

Mr D. sat quietly for a minute and said that he had not been moved by my 'little speech'. He then returned to his silence for about five minutes. I then said I thought that what had just happened between us must reflect something basic to his experience. I had felt sadness, part of which was no doubt my own, something attributable to my own sense of extreme loneliness in being with him. I added that none the less I felt that in part I was feeling something for him, in his stead. I said that I had in the past tried to talk with him about it, but that his replies had always made me feel as if I were either crazy or stupid or both. I said that if I were not in a position to feel some confidence in my ability to differentiate between what feels real and what does not, I would find it a great strain to have my perceptions called into question in such a fundamental way. I told him that it would surprise me greatly if at important points in his life, he had not felt this type of strain in relation to his own ability to differentiate which parts of his experience and perceptions were real and which were not. It seemed from my experience in being with him that he must have felt powerfully assaulted in his efforts to hold on to a conviction about the truth of what he thought, saw, felt, heard and so on.

The patient seemed to ignore almost all of what I had just said and instead commented that I had used the word 'brutalised' in our first meeting. That word was the most accurate word, and 'maybe the only accurate word' that I had used in all these months of analysis. He said that he had never been beaten or abused as a child, but he had felt that he had been brutalised in subtle and in not so subtle ways that he could not describe because he was not even sure what occurred, if in fact anything out of the ordinary did occur. Mr D. said that he would not try to tell me about his childhood because it was all very normal: 'I've gone over it a hundred times with my previous analysts and there isn't anything that would earn me a place on the *Donahue Show.*'

This exchange was the closest Mr D. and I had come to talking to one another. Over the next several weeks, he became increasingly antagonistic and disparaging of me and the analysis. I interpreted the fact that his attacks on me and our efforts to talk to one another had increased dramatically after the meeting that I have just described. At one point, the patient expressed great contempt for my use of the word 'work' to describe what was occurring in these 'very expensive hours'. I said to Mr D. that earlier he had commented on my use of another word, the word 'brutalised'. I told him that I thought that his having acknowledged feeling understood by me, if only in my use of that single word, had led him to feel that things between the two of us had become wildly and dangerously out of control. I said that I thought that what currently appeared on the surface to be his brutalising me, felt to me more like an effort to protect me by getting me to throw him out. I added that I suspected that if I did not soon terminate our meetings he would end the analysis as the only way he felt he had at his disposal to protect me from what he feared to be his endlessly escalating brutalisation of me. Mr D. did not end the analysis, but for a period of almost six months he turned his chair at the beginning of the meeting so that his back was to me. I suspect that he did not want me to be able to see his eyes. In that phase of work, he spoke even less than in the initial months of analysis.

In the portion of the analysis discussed above, Mr D. had in fantasy put into me the fragile remainder of his sense of life and hope. I was to speak for him and feel for him (by beginning each meeting and by being the container of his projective identifications involving his profound loneliness and sadness) while he attacked me for being so naïve as to imagine that I could safeguard his life and my own in the face of his immense brutality. Extreme splitting of the brutalised and brutalising aspects of the patient had been a necessary condition for any form of relatedness to me to be sustained. In the course of the analysis, the patient began to experience for himself the rudiments of sadness and compassion for the aspects of himself which he had projected into me and had experienced through me.

III

In ongoing consultation with clinicians who come to me to discuss analyses that they are conducting, I ask that the analyst attempt to talk with me not only about what the analyst and analysand say to one another, but also about the analyst's moment-to-moment thoughts, feelings and sensations. The analyst is asked to include this aspect of his work in his process notes that he records during the analytic hours and discusses with me in our consultation meetings. In addition, I suggest that the analyst write process notes for all meetings including those that the patient fails to attend. I operate under the assumption that the patient's physical absence creates a specific form of psychological effect in the analyst and in the analysis, and that the analytic process continues despite the analysand's physical absence. In this way, the specific meanings of the patient's presence in his absence are transformed into analytic objects to be fully experienced, lived with, symbolised, understood and made part of the analytic discourse.

In using process notes in this way, the analyst attempts to symbolise and speak to himself about his experience with the patient no matter how seemingly unrelated to the analysand, the analyst's fantasies, physical sensations, ruminations, daydreams, and so on might appear to be (Ogden, 1992a, b, 1994a, b, c, d). I do not 'insist' that a supervisee discuss with me this aspect of the analytic experience since some analysts are initially temperamentally incapable of attending to this level of their experience. Moreover, the analysts consulting with me are not always sufficiently at ease with themselves or with me to entrust this aspect of their work to me. However, I have found that as the supervisory relationship unfolds, supervisees are usually able to develop these capabilities and make use of this aspect of the analytic experience in their therapeutic work and in consultation. I have also found that it is rare for a therapist to be able to engage in this form of supervisory experience without having previously taken part in a successful personal analysis. In the absence of such an experience in analysis (which is not to invoke the illusion of the 'completed analysis'), it is unusual for a therapist to have developed the capacity to make analytic use of his mundane, quotidian, unobtrusive thoughts, feelings and sensations that occupy him during the analytic hours.

As with most aspects of analytic technique, attention to and use of the analyst's private discourse that is seemingly unrelated to the patient run counter to the character defences that we have developed in the course of our lives. To attempt to loosen our dependence on these character defences often feels like 'tearing off a layer of skin', leaving us with a diminished stimulus barrier with which to protect the boundary between inner and outer, between receptivity and over-stimulation, between sanity and insanity.

The analytic work that I shall now describe occurred in the context of the supervision of an analyst who had been consulting with me on a weekly basis for about a year. The analysis had begun in a way that was quite disappointing to the analyst. The analysand, Dr C., was a resident in family practice medicine who had read about psychoanalysis in college, medical school and residency. He had a strong sense of the 'rules of analysis' and complied with them, although from the beginning he complained about the rigidity of the 'game', e.g. the analysand's having to pay for missed meetings, the 'requirement' that the analysand take his vacations when the analyst does, the demand for compliance with the 'fundamental rule', etc. (With the exception of the fee arrangement, the analyst had said nothing about these 'rules'.)

Dr C.'s reasons for being in analysis were vague: he felt he should 'learn about himself' as part of his training as a family practice physician. The idea that he was asking for help with the psychological pain that he was experiencing would have represented an imagined act of submission that the patient could not have tolerated at the beginning of the analysis. The analysand was on time for each session and compliantly 'free associated', presenting a blend of dreams, childhood memories, sexual fantasies and current work-related, marital and child-rearing difficulties and stresses. There were confessions of secret acts about which the patient felt shame, for example, the use of pornographic magazines during masturbation and two incidents of cheating on medical school laboratory reports.

However, from the earliest days and weeks of analysis, the analyst, Dr F., experienced the patient as boring to a degree to which he was unaccustomed. It felt as if the patient were attempting to imitate what he had imagined went on in a 'good analysis'. It required considerable forbearance for Dr F. to refrain from entering into the analysis with interpretations of the content that was being presented, for example, interpretation of dream material that 'seemed to beg for transference interpretations'. In consultation, Dr F. discussed the possible interpretations that he might have made, but had chosen to defer. It seemed to me that these interpretations would have been imitations of 'deep' transference interpretations and would have been offered in an effort on the part of Dr F. to create his own fantasy of a 'good analysis'. As time went on, the analyst felt greatly tempted to chastise the analysand or even comment contemptuously on the emptiness of the patient's verbiage. At each stage, an important perspective that was elaborated in the consultation included the idea that it was of critical importance for Dr F. not to enter into an empty (inert) discourse with the patient and at the same time it was crucial that the analyst maintain his capacity to entertain any thought, feeling, or sensation that arose within him (see Bion, 1978; Symington, 1983). No possible interpretation or response to the patient was to be reflexively dismissed or stifled. It required enormous psychological discipline on the part of Dr F. to resist becoming mechanical, detached or imitative of an idealised version of his own analyst or of me.

Dr F. developed his own style of taking process notes in which he was able to capture something of the totality of the experience of the hour, including the details of his own experience. I think of this as the effort of the analyst to focus upon the countertransference aspects of the transference–countertransference as 'total situation' (Joseph, 1985; Klein, 1952; Ogden, 1991). In other words, it is the transference–countertransference, not simply the transference, that constitutes the matrix in which psychological meanings are generated in the analytic situation.

As Dr F. presented the hours to me in our weekly consultation sessions, neither of us felt pressured to draw one-to-one correspondences between Dr F.'s thoughts and feelings and those of the patient. At times, we each offered tentative understandings of the relationship between Dr F.'s experience and what was happening in the analytic hour. Usually, Dr F.'s reveries were simply noted and were allowed to reverberate within him and me as we listened to the subsequent material. We sometimes referred back in our discussions to reveries that Dr F. had presented in consultation meetings weeks or months earlier.

Dr F.'s thoughts in the initial months of analysis often included wishful images of his upcoming vacations or memories of recent browsing in interesting shops and bookstores during his afternoon breaks. These were understood not simply as generic escapist fantasies, but in each instance were felt to reflect a specific response to what was occurring in the analysis at that particular moment. At one point, several of Dr F.'s vacation daydreams were of an unrealistically idealised sort and seemed to reflect the make-believe nature of the analysis. The patient did not want an actual analysis, he defensively desired a perfect one. In other words, the analysand unconsciously wished for an omnipotently created analysis that did not involve actual encounters between himself and another person with all the anxieties associated with the human lapses, misunderstandings and so on that that would have entailed.

Dr F. attempted to keep alive in himself his capacity to be curious, to question, to comment spontaneously on what was occurring in the analytic interaction despite the 'canned' responses that he would often receive from the patient. 'Analytic etiquette' was not treated as sacred by Dr F., much to the patient's surprise and disapproval. For instance, the patient at one point indicated that he wanted advice from Dr F., but immediately added that he knew that Dr F. could not give him advice. Dr F. responded by asking the patient why he could not give the patient advice. In the end, no advice was given, and instead there was a discussion of the patient's use of fantasised rules (his own omnipotent creations and projections) for the purpose of preventing himself from experiencing and thinking about the personal, idiosyncratic, unpredictable nature of the experience that was occurring between himself and Dr F.

When Dr F. found himself feeling curious about an aspect of the material that the patient was discussing, he asked the patient for further details even when the questions seemed tangential. For example, at one point, Dr F. asked the patient for the name of a restaurant that the patient had parenthetically mentioned having enjoyed the previous evening. The analyst was well aware that the omission of the detail (the name of the restaurant) very likely represented a way of tantalising and excluding the analyst (a projection of the patient's curiosity and feeling of exclusion from the life of the analyst). However, at the time, Dr F. decided to ask (perhaps more accurately, found himself asking) for the detail about which he felt curious while deferring exploration of the tantalising effect of the omission of this particular detail. Coltart (1986) has made a similar recommendation with regard to allowing oneself to laugh at a patient's jokes before analysing the conscious and unconscious motivations of the patient's wish to get the analyst to laugh.

It should be emphasised that while Dr F. attempted to ensure space in the analysis for spontaneity and 'freedom of thought', he by no means treated the analytic frame in a cavalier way – hours were begun and ended in a timely way; casual conversation did not occur between the waiting room and the consulting room; suggestion, reassurance, exhortation, and the like played no larger a part in this analysis than in others conducted by this careful and thoughtful analyst.

For most of the first year of analysis, Dr F. felt that the life of the analysis resided almost entirely in his own capacity to maintain his freedom for reverie during the analytic hours and in his discussions with me of these reveries. By the beginning of the first half of the second year of analysis, the patient began to evidence changes in his ability to speak with a voice of his own that no longer seemed quite as clichéd, stereotyped and imitative as before. However, the changes seemed fragile and short-lived to Dr F.

In this period of the analysis, Dr F. presented a session in consultation in which the patient was silent for the first few minutes of the meeting. Dr F. told me that during this period of silence he had been thinking about the fact that I would be spending my Christmas break in Hawaii. He wondered if I would bring Christmas presents along with me on the trip, all wrapped in shiny red and green paper. He imagined how odd it would be to exchange Christmas gifts in Hawaii and pictured my wife giving me a woollen sweater as a Christmas gift. I commented that I thought Dr F. was expressing scepticism about some of the ideas that we had been discussing in the course of the supervision, particularly the emphasis I had been placing on the importance of Dr F.'s capacity for creativity and spontaneity in his work (as opposed to adopting reflexive, imitative, pre-fabricated approaches).

In the course of discussing Dr F.'s reverie concerning my vacation, I said to Dr F. that I thought that he was depicting me as participating in a self-deceptive charade in which I was treating Christmas as something that could be dug up and moved from one place to another without any change in the experience, just as one might move a plant from one side of a garden to another. The feeling in the daydream was that Christmas had become entirely a form for me and that I had lost touch with any meaning or feeling beyond the stereotypic form. This reverie depicted Dr F.'s disappointment, as well as some degree of competitive pleasure, in viewing me as lacking self-understanding with regard to my own mechanicalness.

It seemed to both Dr F. and to me that Dr F. was saying to both of us, 'Ogden talks a good game about realness, authenticity, genuineness, spontaneity, and so on, but when it comes down to it, maybe he doesn't know what's real and what isn't.' Dr F. and I discussed the way in which my placing a premium on spontaneity may have created a dilemma of sorts for Dr F.: he may have begun to find himself attempting to 'train himself' to be spontaneous. To make matters worse, he may have unconsciously felt that 'achieving spontaneity' would involve imitating me. Dr F. came to see more clearly, as a result of the discussion of this Christmas reverie, that his patient had been labouring under a similar burden in the analysis for some time. For months, Dr C. had said that he felt an internal pressure to be 'on' in analysis, that is, to be interesting to Dr F. Only at this point did Dr C.'s comment take on an analytic meaning (become an 'analytic object') that could be symbolised, reflected upon and interpreted. Dr F. felt that he now better understood that the patient's internal pressure to be 'on' reflected the patient's unconscious fantasy that he could only be alive for Dr F. to the degree that he could learn to think, feel, speak, and behave in a manner like or the same as Dr F. This placed the patient in an impossible position in which feeling alive and being interesting to Dr F. had become synonymous. Paradoxically, the idea of feeling alive had for Dr C. become unconsciously equivalent to becoming (an idealised version of) Dr F.

In the course of the succeeding weeks of analysis, Dr F. offered to the analysand his understanding of this dilemma that he believed to underlie Dr C.'s feeling of pressure to be 'on' in analysis. Both this interpretation and Dr F.'s self-understanding upon which it rested facilitated the creation of psychological space in the analysis in which both the patient and analyst were able to continue to develop their capacity to generate thoughts, feelings and sensations without feeling that there was an unstated script or paradigm that either of them was being asked to mouth or imitate.

In the clinical sequence just described, it was essential for the analyst to be able to have his own thoughts independent of mine (which need was symbolised by Dr F.'s unconscious criticism of me in the Christmas reverie). Only when Dr F. became aware of the way in which his own capacity for original thought had been paralysed by his fear of confronting his defensive idealisation of me, could he regain his full capacity for reverie. Dr F.'s symbolisation of, and understanding of, this defensive process as it was portrayed in the Christmas reverie formed the basis for his interpretation of his patient's futile attempts to overcome his own experience of deadness by (in fantasy) attempting to become a perfect patient, that is, to become a defensively idealised version of his conception of an analytic patient.

IV

The final clinical vignette that I shall present will focus on the problem of 'competing' (Tustin, 1980; see also Ogden, 1989a, b) with a form of deadness that involves a pathologically autistic aspect of personality. In the analysis of adult patients, the autistic component of the personality is often not at all evident in the beginning of analysis (S. Klein, 1980). This was the case in the analysis of Mrs S. In the initial analytic meeting, Mrs S. talked about her difficulties in 'getting her life together'. She had not been able to graduate from college as a result of her inability to concentrate. Her marriage was in disarray and she felt on the edge of panic.

It is not possible in the space of the present chapter to offer an account of the stages of the evolution of the analytic process over the first eight years of this five session per week analysis. The outcome of these years of work might be very broadly summarised by saying that despite the fact that there had been important changes in the patient's ability to function in the world (for example, she was able to graduate from college and hold a responsible job), the patient's capacity to enter into relationships with other people remained very limited. Mrs S. and her husband slept in separate bedrooms and on occasion engaged in what the patient described as 'mechanical sex'. It had required more than five years of analysis for the patient to even recognise that she 'managed' her three children as if she were 'an employee of a day-care centre' and that she had very little sense of each of them as individuals. Her friendships were shallow and only toward the end of the seventh year of analysis did she begin to feel the absence of loving relationships in her life.

In the analytic relationship, I was again and again stunned (in a way that I have rarely experienced with other patients) by the depth of the patient's inability to evidence or experience any warmth toward me. It was not that Mrs S. did not feel dependent on me. She was greatly distressed by weekend breaks, vacations (her own as well as mine), the end of each session, and would frequently telephone my answering machine in order to hear my voice (without leaving a message of her own). However, Mrs S. experienced her dependence not as a personal attachment, but as an addiction that she deeply resented: 'A heroin addict does not love heroin. The fact that she'll kill to get it doesn't mean she loves it or feels any kind of affection for it.' The patient felt powerfully untouchable in her isolation and seemed to value this feeling of 'being immune to human vulnerabilities' more than anything else in life. This 'untouchable' quality was reflected in her anorectic symptomatology. The patient subsisted on a diet of fruit, grains and vegetables and organised her life around a rigorous exercise regime that included marathon jogging and the extensive use of a stationary bicycle. The patient exercised vigorously for at least three hours every day. If the exercise routine were in any way disrupted (for example, by illness or by travel), the patient would experience a state of intense anxiety that on two occasions developed into full-blown panic attacks. Mrs S., at the beginning of the analysis experienced no appetite for food, sex, ideas, art or anything else. The patient's weight held the greatest importance for her: by maintaining a particular weight (at the very low end of what she could tolerate physiologically without falling physically ill), she experienced a form of power that allowed her in fantasy to control everything that might occur both within her and outside of her.

It would be inaccurate to say that the patient always felt numb or without feelings in the analytic hours. Mrs S. frequently experienced intense anger, which she called 'hatred', towards me. However, her anger never seemed personal. By this I mean that it never felt as if her anger had anything to do with me. The hatred did not even seem to be the patient's personal creation; rather, it seemed like a blind, reflexive, almost convulsive thrashing about that occurred when her sense of absolute control and ownership of me was compromised. Since I was the person/object who happened to be there, it was I who happened to be the object of her rage. Mrs S.'s criticism of me always involved her projective fantasy of my omnipotence: she felt that I could easily give her what she needed if I chose to, but that I stubbornly refused to do so.

Other than her single-minded crusade to gain access to my fantasised omnipotent power, there seemed to be very little about me that was of interest to the patient. It was difficult for me to accept how little I seemed to mean to this patient outside of the terms of the fantasy I am discussing. For years, I held to the belief that Mrs S. secretly loved me (albeit in a primitive way), felt a form of concern for me, knew something about who I am as a person, but stubbornly refused to admit it. This belief was based on the intensity of the patient's feeling of dependence on me in conjunction with the fact that I felt concern for and interest in her. At times, I interpreted what I felt to be the patient's anxiety about acknowledging any feeling of human connection with me for fear of the loss of control over her external and internal world that that would entail. She would respond by saying that what I said might be true, but she was not aware of feeling affection, love, warmth or even concern for me or for anyone else for that matter. The defensive function of such a stance on the patient's part was discussed on many occasions, but did not lead to any discernible affective change. (These interpretations felt increasingly stale to both the patient and to me.)

Perhaps it was the patient's response to the death of my father that was the beginning of my loosening of my hold on the belief that the patient secretly felt some form of love or concern for me. The events transpiring between Mrs S. and myself around this event (in the eighth year of analysis) led me to feel that there was a qualitative difference between the human disconnectedness achieved by Mrs S. and forms of defence against the dangers of love and hate that I had encountered with other patients. After receiving the unexpected news of my father's death, I telephoned my patients and supervisees to tell them that there had been a death in my family and that I would be cancelling several days' meetings. I told each of them that I would phone them to tell them when I would be resuming work. When I spoke with Mrs S., she received the news quietly, but immediately asked me if I knew approximately when I would be returning to work. I said that I did not know, but would let her know when I did.

In our first meeting after my return, Mrs S. said that she was 'sorry that someone in my family had died'. There was unmistakable anger in her voice as she underscored the vagueness of the word 'someone'. She fell silent for a few minutes and then said that it made her feel furious not to know who it was that had died and said that she felt that I had been sadistic in not giving her that information when I phoned her. She added that she was certain that I had told all my other patients who it was in my family that had died. During this interchange, I felt deeply disturbed by a recognition against which I had struggled for most of a decade: it seemed to me that Mrs S. was unable to feel anything for me as a human being beyond her need to protect herself by means of her efforts to magically enter me and control me from within.

At this point in the meeting, I began to recall the details of the feelings that I had experienced during the telephone call that I had made to Mrs S. soon after I learned of my father's death. I remembered with great vividness the feeling of attempting to control my voice as I spoke to her in an effort to hold back tears. I wondered whether it was possible that she registered nothing of that. How could she have not experienced that moment (as I had) as one in which there had been a close connection between the two of us? Instead, she apparently experienced it as still another occasion in which her omnipotent wishes had been frustrated.

I could hear the voice with which I was speaking to myself at that moment in the meeting as the voice of a person experiencing a sense of impenetrable alienation from Mrs S.; at the same time, I also recognised something else in that voice for the first time. It was the voice of a spurned lover. It occurred to me that Mrs S. lived in a world in which two different forms of human experience each disguised the other.

At that juncture, I felt that I had arrived at the beginnings of an understanding of something about the relationship between Mrs S. and myself that I had not previously grasped. This new understanding did not serve to protect me from the chilling inhumanness that I had sensed in Mrs S. and which I knew reflected important autistic and paranoid-schizoid elements in her personality; neither did it serve to dim the recognition that alongside these powerful autistic and paranoid-schizoid defences was a capacity for human love. I could at this point see in retrospect that it was in part my own lack of compassion for Mrs S. and her wishes to comfort me *as my wife* that had led me to blind myself to the fact that her seeming absence of compassion represented a complex interplay of two powerful, coexisting aspects of her personality. She had been concerned about me and felt despondent that her love was unrecognisable to me (for example, as reflected in my not allowing her to comfort me). At the same time there was an important way in which Mrs S. was unable to come to life as a human being and instead occupied a mechanical, omnipotent world of: (1) relatedness to 'autistic shapes' and 'autistic objects' (Tustin, 1980, 1984) (for example, the mechanical, self-sufficiency involved in the sensation-world of exercise and diet), and (2) paranoid-schizoid fantasies of entering me and parasitically living in me and through me.

I had been unable to live with, formulate and interpret for myself and for the patient the mutually obscuring interrelationship between being alive and being dead (i. e. the coexistence of depressive, paranoid-schizoid and autistic-contiguous (Ogden, 1989 a, b) dimensions of the patient's personality). Mrs S. had loved me and had felt nothing whatever for me at the same time. I had experienced affection for her (which I came to recognise more fully in my experience of feeling like a spurned lover), but could not allow myself to feel warmth or at times even feel compassion for someone who was so clearly inhuman and inhumane (for example, in her treatment of her husband, her children and in her response to me, particularly after my father's death).

Later in the session that I am describing, I said to Mrs S. that I thought I had underestimated two things in our relationship: the amount of affection that there was and the degree to which no relationship at all existed between us. When I lost sight of one or the other facet of the situation, I failed to understand the totality of who she is and who we are together. I added that I thought that the degree to which it was possible for there to be no human tie between us had diminished in the time that we had known one another, but that it remained a considerable force to be reckoned with.

Mrs S. responded by saying that I had never spoken to her in that way before. Previously, she had always felt that there was a way in which I was as cold as she was and that she could hear that iciness in my voice. She could not detect that coldness in me just now. Mrs S. went on to say that she did not believe that that iciness was gone, but at least it did not dominate everything that occurred between us for the moment.

I understood this to be a statement of the patient's feeling of relief at her sense that she could accept understanding from me, which was something she had never before been able to do without immediately attacking it, or more often, withdrawing into a state of autistic self-sufficiency or omnipotent paranoid-schizoid defensive fantasy. My interpretation had denied neither her emotional deadness (her paranoid-schizoid and autistic-contiguous modes of protecting herself) nor her increased capacity to experience a human connection to me (albeit very sparingly acknowledged by her).

Concluding comments

Four clinical discussions have been presented in an effort to illustrate ways in which the sense of aliveness and deadness are generated and experienced in and through the intersubjective analytic third. In each of the clinical situations described, the analyst attempted to create analytic meaning ('analytic objects') from that which had been unconsciously present, and powerfully shaping of the analytic encounter, but had been foreclosed from the analytic discourse. It was through the analyst's use of his reveries, his unobtrusive, quotidian, thoughts, feelings and sensations (often seemingly unrelated to the patient) that specific, verbally symbolised meanings were generated and eventually utilised in the interpretative process. In the four analyses described, the particular quality of the experience of aliveness and deadness generated in the transference–countertransference constituted an important intersubjective construction that reflected a central aspect of the analysand's pathologically structured internal object world.

© The Institute of Psycho-Analysis

Note

1   I use the term *countertransference* to refer to the analyst's experience of and contribution to the transference–countertransference. The latter term refers to an unconscious intersubjective construction generated by the analytic pair. I do not view transference and countertransference as separable entities that arise in response to one another; rather, I understand these terms to refer to aspects of a

single intersubjective totality experienced separately (and individually) by analyst and analysand.

References

Bion, W. R. (1959) Attacks on linking. *International Journal of Psycho-Analysis* 40: 308–15.

—— (1962) *Learning from Experience.* New York: Basic Books.

—— (1978) *Four Discussions with W. R. Bion.* Perthshire: Clunie Press.

Bollas, C. (1987) *The Shadow of the Object: Psychoanalysis of the Unthought Known.* New York: Columbia University Press.

Casement, P. (1985) *Learning from the Patient.* New York: Guilford.

Coltart, N. (1986) Slouching towards Bethlehem ... or thinking the unthinkable in psychoanalysis. In G. Kohon (ed.) *The British School of Psychoanalysis: The Independent Tradition.* New Haven, CT: Yale University Press. (Also in N. Coltart (1992). *Slouching towards Bethlehem ... and Further Psychoanalytic Explorations.* London: FAB.)

Green, A. (1975) The analyst, symbolization and absence in the analytic setting (On changes in analytic practice and analytic experience). *International Journal of Psycho-Analysis* 56: 1–22.

—— (1983) The dead mother. In *On Private Madness.* Madison, CT: International Universities Press, 1986.

Joseph, B. (1985) Transference: the total situation. *International Journal of Psycho-Analysis* 66: 447–54.

Klein, M. (1952) The origins of transference. In *Envy and Gratitude and Other Works, 1946–1963.* New York: Delacorte.

Klein, S. (1980) Autistic phenomena in neurotic patients. *International Journal of Psycho-Analysis* 61: 395–401.

Meares, R. (1993) *The Metaphor of Play.* Northvale, NJ: Jason Aronson.

Mitchell, S. (1993) *Hope and Dread in Psychoanalysis.* New York: Basic Books.

Ogden, T. (1989a) On the concept of an autistic-contiguous position. *International Journal of Psycho-Analysis* 70: 127–40.

—— (1989b) *The Primitive Edge of Experience.* Northvale, NJ: Jason Aronson.

—— (1991) Analysing the matrix of transference. *International Journal of Psycho-Analysis* 72: 593–605.

—— (1992a) The dialectically constituted/decentred subject of psychoanalysis. I. The Freudian subject. *International Journal of Psycho-Analysis* 73: 517–26.

—— (1992b) The dialectically constituted/decentred subject of psychoanalysis. II. The contributions of Klein and Winnicott. *International Journal of Psycho-Analysis* 73: 613–26.

——. (1994a) The analytic third – working with intersubjective clinical facts. *International Journal of Psycho-Analysis* 75: 3–20.

—— (1994b) The concept of interpretative action. *Psychoanalytic Quarterly* 63: 219–45.

—— (1994c) Identifição projetiva e o terceiro subjugador. *Revista de Psicanílise de Sociedade Psicanalítica de Porto Alegre* 2: 153–62. (Published in English as 'Projective identification and the subjugating third'. In *Subjects of Analysis.* Northvale, NJ: Jason Aronson.)

—— (1994d) *Subjects of Analysis*. Northvale, NJ: Jason Aronson.

Stewart, H. (1977) Problems of management in the analysis of a hallucinating hysteric. *International Journal of Psycho-Analysis* 38: 67–76.

Symington, N. (1983) The analyst's act of freedom as agent of therapeutic change. *International Review of Psycho-Analysis* 10: 283–91. Also in G. Kohon (ed.) *The British School of Psychoanalysis: The Independent Tradition*. New Haven, CT: Yale University Press, 1986.

Tustin, F. (1980) Autistic objects. *International Review of Psycho-Analysis* 7: 27–40.

Tustin, S. (1984) Autistic shapes. *International Review of Psycho-Analysis* 11: 279–90.

Winnicott, D. W. (1951) Transitional objects and transitional phenomena. In *Playing and Reality*. New York: Basic Books.

—— (1971) The place where we live. In *Playing and Reality*. NewYork: Basic Books.

7

THE DEAD MOTHER

Variations on a theme

André Lussier

André Green's masterful study of the psychodynamic consequences of the mother's psychological death in the early years of life has become an indispensable source of inspiration for any work dealing with related clinical psychodynamics. The present chapter is meant as a tribute, and a testimony to my clinical and theoretical indebtedness towards André Green.

In his paper, Green described and analysed the many layers that had to be peeled off, one by one, during the psychoanalysis of male and female patients suffering the psychological loss of the mother early in life – a mother still alive, but emotionally unavailable to the child owing to sudden depression caused by a severe loss. The analysis proceeds from the most superficial layers to the very deep. Initial work on the characterological depressive structure, for instance, will expose a depression with many faces or meanings; the patient feels depressed but for a long time remains unaware of his unconscious identification with his depressed mother – his only way of keeping her alive, buried so to speak within himself. In the final stages, the analysis reveals a deep-seated longing for the ideal loving mother, the good mother that preceded the depressed one, and Green elaborates on the refusal to give up and mourn this ideal mother.

A major role is thus ascribed to the mechanism of unconscious identification as a way of keeping the love object inside when there is a great threat of loss. All this is perfectly consistent with some of Freud's views on the psychodynamics of depression (Freud, 1917), even though, as Green informs us, we are not dealing with classical depression in this case. Putting the focus on identification greatly appeals to me and in this chapter I want to make it the centre of my reflection. I will discuss two types of patients: first a group of female patients, followed by a group of male patients, all of whom suffered the psychological loss, i.e. the symbolic death, of a parent at an early age, and for whom this loss represents the first (known) and most determining trauma in the history of their neurosis.

I intend to focus on the significant similarities and dissimilarities between my patients and those of Green. On the whole I would say that, despite obvious dissimilarities, all the patients involved belong to the same category of psychopathology. My patients represent variations on Green's theme of the dead mother. With the group of female patients, the significant trauma was the psychological loss of the mother between the ages of two and three; in contrast, the male patients' trauma was the psychological loss of the father between the ages of three and six. It might appear strange to include patients suffering from the emotional loss of their father in a paper honouring 'The dead mother', but, as psychoanalysts, we are mainly interested in the working of unconscious mechanisms and thought processes in analogous situations, and this is the case with the loss of the father.

Female patients

Like Green's patients, these women did not seek analysis because of depression but because of characterological problems, in particular the difficulty of sustaining a loving relationship with a man. They considered themselves responsible for these repeated failures, becoming almost phobic as soon as a relationship with a man grew more intimate and serious.

The mother as terror

Many years of analysis have shown that these women, unlike Green's patients, did not seem to experience the mother as depressed either immediately following the early trauma suffered by mother and child (i.e. tragic divorce with permanent loss of the father, death of the father through road accident), or long afterwards. However, the mothers appeared depressed late in life, managing to induce their daughters (my patients as adults) to act as mothers, mothering their own mother. The most astonishing characteristic of the childhood years, dramatically exposed only late in the analysis, was that, at first the mothers appeared angry right from the time of the trauma, being aggressively hostile towards their daughter, frighteningly rejecting, neglectful, and utterly controlling to a sadistic degree. Even though this should be seen as centrally determining in the emotional life of the patients, it must be emphasised that it took many years of laborious analysis to uncover it with certainty. The psychological fact is that this terrifying attitude of the mother was 'successfully' covered up by a massive arsenal of defensive measures initiated by denial and idealisation. It will be shown that we are not dealing here with the denial of a depression affecting the mother but rather with the denial by the child of the mother's terrifying hostility. (One could also speak in terms of denial of depression, but only in so far as the depression of the child is concerned.)

Though heavily resorting to denial, these patients gave plenty of evidence that this mechanism was a very fragile protection; it had to be continuously supported and reinforced, along with other defences, by a specific life-long behavioural and mental complex destined to counter the dreadful unconscious truth. I could summarise a major portion of these analyses and of the life of these patients in the following condensed formulas: it is not true that my mother hated me, she felt nothing but love for me; it is not true that I was full of rage against her, I had only love for her. Such deceptively simple statements necessitated a huge amount of work in analysis before they could emerge as a naked truth. This struggle for life, for love, in some respects, was acted out on two fronts: directly with their real mothers and indirectly, but powerfully, through a compulsive type of object relationships with female friends. Both of these elements affected the transference and the counter-transference. At this point of my exposé, I will concentrate on the actual relationship to the real mother; I will return to the topic of the female friends further on.

Life-long mother–child relationship

From the start, the relationship with the mother, replete with denial, drew the analyst's attention. If one keeps in mind that we are dealing with women well within the range of psychological 'normalcy' (i.e. not pathologically regressed), functioning well professionally, and aged between 30 and 50, what follows is astonishing. During the analysis, every week if not several times a week, these adult women felt compelled to call their mother in order to remind her of their love, and in the futile hope of hearing their declaration reciprocated. It was repetitive: 'I called my mother just to tell her, *I love you.*' The disappointing lack of reciprocity never altered the pattern. When the patients were sick, they also called their mothers in the hope of getting some comforting words of sympathy, once again in vain. The mothers were not interested and quickly changed the topic of conversation, in order to focus on themselves only; the habit nevertheless persisted. Similarly, the patients paid regular weekly visits to their mothers with the same obstinate purpose, namely to attest their 'unfailing' love. These women were compelled all their life to prove that they still were 'good girls'.

At one point, the analyst began to realise that these rather compulsive habits were being reinforced as the analysis progressed, and this gave rise to counter-transferential reactions. It all started with my feeling that the repetition of these habits was gradually fulfilling a transferential function; appearing increasingly as a defiance of the analyst, it clearly became a challenge to the analytical work. One could well surmise that, sooner or later, the analysis would be experienced as a threat to the maintenance of the beliefs and habits in question. The patients started in earnest unconsciously to protect themselves against the danger of uncovering the false love and the false-self, fighting desperately to avoid the confrontation with the unbearable truth of not being loved when there is no father to resort to. That these mothers were anything but loving after the trauma was something soon to be evident to the analyst. With each renewed affirmation of the belief in reciprocal love, the denial, the reaction formation and the mini-delusion (Winnicott) were becoming transparent. Gradually, the pseudo love-relationship started to come apart and to crumble for the patient, a process which was utterly painful throughout. The dual transference–countertransference relationship was the first scene of action where the transformation could be experienced in distress. The patients accused the analyst of being an 'enemy', referring to his disbelief when they were talking about their love for their mothers or their mother's love for them. The analyst had to proceed with special care due to the fact that some of these accusations were indeed well founded, and it became a delicate operation to work upon the still heavy projection on the part of the patients.

Several times during this process, one patient, more sensitive to the deep distress she anticipated, did exclaim: 'I cannot, I am not able not to go visiting my mother regularly, I cannot', as if to say: 'don't force me, it is beyond me'. Later on, she declared: 'the day I stop visiting my mother to prove my love, I will be cured'.

Today, I could say unequivocally that it gradually dawned on the patients that they were projecting onto the analyst the attitude that, from early childhood on, they had been too terrified to assume. It was there, none the less, inside, deeply repressed, and it was finally coming out into the open as projected onto the analyst. As an 'enemy', professing his disbelief of love, he was a thorough projection of an unconscious self-image, the image of the hostile child they so feared being made aware of. Uncovering the disbelief unavoidably meant loosening up hostility and rage against the mother. André Green spoke of the buried depressed mother, deeply introjected and identified with; I could speak, in a parallel way, of the buried self-image of the angry child, a powerfully guarded image, enveloped by layers of defensive measures.

Why is it that these patients had to be so desperately defensive with regard to any sign of hostility and anger? I would simply say that it was in order to avoid at all cost the catastrophe of deep depression. After the traumatic experience of losing the father, the mother is the only surviving parental figure: if, at that point, the child unleashes the hostile raging and destructive feelings against the unloving mother, they may well anticipate falling into the abyss of an empty world. The child is facing two catastrophes: the unassimilable awareness of not being loved, and the awful anticipation of an empty world.

Blank depression

When the first cracks appeared in the defensive delusional organisation of my patients, heavy depressive feelings started to take over. As I said before, there was no sign of identification with a depressed mother and, truly, I was prepared for it, having read Green several times. However, in another theoretical respect, Green's general views on depression could provide a basis for understanding my patients' form of depression. The psychodynamics of these patients, when depressed, did not correspond to the classical picture of a regressed cruel superego, sadistically crushing a powerless and guilty ego identified with the lost love-object. Green's views are relevant here. He describes another type of depression, blank depression, which he considers as deeper than the 'black' one. The devastating factor here is not caused by the manoeuvres of a sadistic superego but rather by the affective workings of the feeling of emptiness, emptiness inside, emptiness outside. Blank depression reveals the inner action of the dread of nothingness, the panic over the feeling of falling into the abyss of a world either without love or without love-objects. It means the threat of total abandonment. My patients, and their unconscious dynamics, fit this model perfectly. Most of their emotional life, their character structure, their object-relationships can be understood as the multifaceted and frantic attempt to counter the threat of emotional abandonment: to deny it, to repress it, to reverse it, to transform it into its opposite, and finally reduce it to silence by building up a mental structure based on mini-delusions.

It may seem puzzling that such a severe depression could be observed in patients who otherwise exhibit the qualities of a relatively sound ego. This corroborates the claim that a relatively well-functioning ego does not necessarily imply an early life devoid of heavy conflicts and traumas. It also suggests that this ego strength must be due to a sound emotional beginning in the mother–child relationship prior to the trauma, in this case before the age of two. The analytic experience has shown in many ways that these patients have been tried to an extreme emotional degree, giving rise at times to the feeling of absolute exhaustion, of being drained by the analysis. I will come back to this point later on while talking about loss of consciousness. It is clear that none of these patients were psychotic to any degree. All of them, though, at times of great despair, when realising how unrealistic their belief in love had been, would declare: 'I must have been insane', while others would say as well: 'Without the analysis, I would have become crazy or I would have committed suicide'. The frontier between the so-called 'normal' and the others is a very thin one. But it appears undeniable that the difference lies in the ego's capacity to withstand and resist the unconscious pressure.

The special identification with the mother

The most meaningful psychic feature of Green's patients was the uncovering of an identification with the depressed mother early in life. Almost everything else revolved around this basic self-representation. With my patients, the similarities and dissimilarities are both worth considering. The main similarity lies in the fact that, in both cases, a deep-seated identification with the mother played a major role in the overall psychic organisation. The object of this identification, however, represents the most fundamental difference: my patients did not identify with a depressed mother after the trauma, but with a sadistically controlling one. In order to assess properly the implications of this feature, one must keep in mind that it took many years of analysis to uncover it.

Late in the analysis, and somewhat suddenly, something thoroughly unexpected happened. These patients were gradually and painfully becoming aware of the shaky foundation of their belief in reciprocal love with their mothers, of the false nature of their obstinate conviction. They witnessed the crumbling of a mental and emotional structure they had strenuously built from early childhood on in order to make life bearable. At that very moment in the analysis, their characterological structure (armour) literally exploded. This paved the way for the appearance (or reappearance?) of a dormant self. On the basis of a global identification with a buried image of the mother, they became abruptly violent, aggressively hostile with their partner in life, sadistically controlling, devastatingly critical and intolerant to an utmost degree. The dramatic impact of these scenes can be grasped if one takes into account that these women, up to that point, considered themselves and were considered by friends and relatives as unfailingly submissive, dependent, non-aggressive and self-controlled, character traits that, of course, betrayed their fragility through their rigidity and compulsiveness. What was now happening to them in reality frightened these women. They felt they were becoming someone else, crazy, possessed. During some of those scenes, while they were sadistically attacking and controlling their spouse in life, what was left of the sound side of their ego permitted some of them to shout to their partner or husband in desperation: 'Please, please stop me, stop me, take me into your arms ...' This vivid image suggests that while the sadistic controlling mother was thoroughly introjected and identified with, more than just being an introject, the internal maternal object remained nevertheless subjected to resistance; either it had not been fully assimilated or the two solutions were kept inside, side by side. The child was too young to be in a psychic condition to resist identifying with the frightening mother – it must have been a sudden and total process; but at the same time, in one little corner of the mind, of the free mind, the child did not welcome this identification with the aggressor. One of the many reasons why the child found this intolerable became clear: it meant the unconscious destruction of the mother, the sole remaining love-object. This deep-seated hostility toward the mother, threatening to destroy her, was one of the main factors pushing the analysand close to the edge of the abyss of nothingness, to the panic of an empty world, of total abandonment, blank depression. During those crucial phases of the analysis, the patients realised clearly enough that they were behaving as though propelled by an identification with their angry mother – they were possessed, as one of them declared.

Reaction to terror

With respect to the possible links between the traumatic experience and the identification with the traumatising aggressor, I was intrigued by the many references to a repeated childhood experience, reported by one patient and corroborated by her relatives. Following the family trauma (divorce and permanent loss of father, angry mother), from the ages of two to four, the little girl lost consciousness on several occasions in the presence of the mother. Because of the timing of allusions to these early events in the analysis, it is plausible to assume that, at the time of the trauma, the child was so frightened by the change in the attitude of the mother, so terrified by her angry impatience, that the only way out was to lose consciousness, thus removing herself from the threatening reality. Absolute denial without psychosis. It appears that the loss of consciousness occurred in a convulsive way. For the reasons already mentioned, the child did not dare react overtly with anger, identifying with the mother; but as an adult, during and because of the analysis, this deep-seated identification burst out into the open, disturbing the conjugal life of her couple. The angry child could take over the passive one. Once again, the context leads me to think that the patient was dealing with an anxiety over extermination or annihilation. Some other phases of the analysis seem to confirm these hypotheses, such as when the most significant factor was another deeply repressed identification: the identification with the dead father (the lost father seen early as chased away and destroyed by the mother). This shows yet another of the severe dilemmas facing the child: either to join in with the mother against the father, or to join in with father against mother (the equivalent of a death wish). I cannot here elaborate on the fact that it seems that the mother, after the trauma of separation, became angry at the father and took the child as victim.

Not only were these repeated experiences of sudden outbursts of angry, hostile behaviour almost unbelievable, they also left the patients prey to depression. The feeling of being possessed led inevitably to the devastating awareness of the mother's angry, hostile character. They found themselves face to face with an unloving mother; it could no longer be denied. The feeling of panic which ensued was as intense as that caused by the phantasy of angrily destroying the only remaining love-object (mother), but it was of a different nature. The unconscious – and now conscious – thoughts involved had a different affect and meaning: essentially the feeling of being nothing. Not being loved means worthlessness: it leaves the child alone with the devastating thought that it is better not to be alive than not being loved. In her superb writings on depression, Edith Jacobson once observed that it is as though the child (destined to become depressed) says to himself: 'It is better to have such a mother – a cruel unloving one – rather than no mother at all.' I would say that it was different with my patients: unable to tolerate the idea of not being loved, they proceeded psychically to replace the actual world (mother) by an imaginary one, thus managing to avoid psychosis.

On the whole, the above considerations help explain the presence of so many layers in the building up of the personality structure of these patients. Unable to tolerate the feeling of being unloved, and equally unable to endure that of being inhabited by a raging love-object, they had to resort extensively to denial, repression, reaction formation, turning into the opposite, and projection. The unloving mother had to be denied any chance of resurfacing. Denial, reaction formation, and turning into the opposite were strenuously activated to transform the mother–child relationship: 'my mother loves me and I love my mother'. As long as that mini-delusion was kept functioning, the identification with the hostile mother remained buried and unthreatening. This brings me back to the high price these patients had to pay in order to maintain their psychic-emotional achievement.

Social relationships

Having explored the semi-delusional and idealised relationship to the mother, I propose now to address another aspect of the high price these women had to pay to preserve their imaginary world. It concerns the nature of their relationships to female friends. They spent the best of their psychic energy establishing these friendships and keeping them at all costs. For them, to live meant having loving female friends and this was achieved in a compulsive and very demanding manner. Strangely enough, it never led, except in dreams, to an open homosexual life, but the language and the affects were identical to the way homosexuals talk about their lovers. With my patients, the female friends had to be as faithful as a lover. Whenever such friends got involved in a heterosexual relationship, my patients would become dramatically jealous and felt deeply betrayed. They could not understand how a real friend could inflict so much pain on them by spending more time with their male friend. They complained of injustice and cruelty. Day after day, they did everything in their power to avoid being alone and feeling lonely. For years, there was not a single session during which they did not talk about the many close female friends with whom they spent their free time. The relationships were described in terms of great intimacy and at times even of fusional togetherness; they represented the only way to make life happy or at least bearable.

I would say that the analysis and the analyst were invaded by a plethora of women, to the extent that they soon developed into a defensive measure against the analytical work. The more these patients felt that the analysis was threatening the relationship to the mother, the more they had to fill the gap with mother substitutes, towards whom they became as demanding as they were towards their own mother. It must be added that the compensatory role played by female friends had begun long before the analysis. Needless to say, these patients proved themselves utterly dependent and submissive with their friends, implying that these relationships were bordering closely on masochism. Their epic determination to save the ties to their 'loving mothers' often meant yielding to domination, exploitation and humiliation. I confess that it was a relief for the analyst when this masochistic trend started to be overcome.

It was again through the transference that a breach began to appear in the compulsive relationships to mother substitutes. They accused the analyst of wanting to deprive them of essential love, to impose a dry ascetic–monastic life. Such transferential episodes in turn helped thrust the patients into a state of dread of abandonment, of panic at the threat of nothingness, of worthlessness, a kind of psychological death. Late in the analysis, terrified of the impending loss of so many needed relationships, they felt again that the world was becoming empty, both outside and inside. These were hours of doom.

As for possible factors involved in preventing the expected outcome (overt homosexuality) from being realised, at the moment I can still venture only one hypothesis based on some manifestations during these analyses, and a rather classical one at that: in spite of the crushing influence of the mother, of the heavy fixation on her, these women reached a minimum degree of triangular investment. In a discreet but sure way, the father and the father-figures were kept alive in the background, so that there was always some hope of getting closer to the father (father-figures). But insecurity prevailed. One of these patients, around the age of twenty, in the very first minutes following her first sexual experience with a man, had anxiously to get up and reach the nearest telephone; she called her mother to tell her that she loved her. All these patients had boyfriends and lovers, but each new heterosexual object relationship generated some level of panic, brought on by the fear that these involvements might cause the loss of their female friends (mother-figures). As expected, this proved to be a repetition of the anxiety they experienced when, as a child, they had good reason to believe that their mother was getting involved with another man.

Mothering men

The third and final life outcome of this early traumatic experience was that, without exception, all the men in their love life had to be primarily mothering figures. During physical intimacy, the sensual manifestations by far outweighed the sexual ones. Sexual intercourse was of little importance. What mattered most was to be touched, to be caressed (but not sexually), to be massaged, to be held. One patient said: 'What I like most with a man is when he accepts to do what my mother never did: to take me in his arms'. With these patients I observed many of the same elements often present in the sexual life of fetishists, namely that in their sexual development, sexuality and its implied triangulation appeared as a *trouble-fête*, a threat to the peaceful, fusional relationship with the mother. One could say that they had one foot in the triangular Oedipal sexual sphere, anxiously poised to retreat.

Male patients

I will be brief about the male patients, focusing on a few themes which reveal a striking similarity with the mental mechanisms analysed by Green in his paper.

Identification with the psychologically dead father

This identification proved to be a forceful structure, strongly resisting psychological change during analysis. As with the female patients, the primary determining factor proved to be the psychological loss of the father early in life (from three to five years of age). Something tragic had happened (to the child) in the course of an initially good relationship to the father: permanent loss through divorce, mental or physical illness.

The analysis made it possible to unravel the many layers of meaning sustaining this identification. One of these meanings seems to belong to the mysterious workings of the 'negative', so acutely analysed by André Green in one of his books: *Le Travail du négatif* (Green, 1993). I refer to the fact that the patients invest negative features (identification with the father as a failure, for instance) for the sake of some underlying narcissistic purpose. This identification with the psychologically 'dead' father manifests itself through specific character traits: passivity, inertia, lack of initiative, inhibition of aggression, dependency, obstinate inclination to rely on a substitute father-figure in the outside world. This last point could serve as an accurate summary of the transference relationship.

The unintrojectable new objects

With some of these patients, the dependence repeatedly took the form of a claim: 'I am entitled to that', referring to a conscious exploitation of the experience of deprivation. I often heard: 'One is entitled to have a father'. This feature is closely related to one of Green's major themes: the failure to introject new objects. During the analysis of these patients, I was amazed by the tenacity of this unique phenomenon. Despite the fact that they encountered in their daily life many highly respected and idealised male figures, the analysis revealed no internal sign that any one of them, the analyst included, had become an introjected good object. Without the slightest hint to that effect from the analyst (as far as one can safely ascertain), some of these patients even became puzzled themselves by the realisation that none of these 'great' men seemed to have retained a significant place in their memory. This alone reveals an uncanny awareness regarding their struggle to keep out any new 'good' object. For many years, I have been trying to understand the mental mechanism at work that Green alludes to when he says *la place est prise*. I describe identical mechanisms in my own patients (in an as yet unpublished paper, presented in Ottawa in 1985), namely that 'there is no room left' for any new introjection: the dead father was filling up the inner space, and the identification with the failing father could not be dislodged. The specific workings of such a mechanism remain a mystery, but at least we have an idea of some of its fundamental underlying purposes. I want to elaborate on this point.

The guardian of the ideal father

The first of these purposes implies a paradox: the firmly entrenched 'dead' father serves as a guardian of another figure, the ideal father himself, even more deeply enshrined as in a crypt (according to the terminology of the French analysts Maria Torok and Nicolas Abraham (1976)). In the analysis of his patients, André Green discovered, concealed behind the introjected dead mother, the sure presence of an ideal mother. Plenty of inner space had been allotted to the dead mother in order to secure the secret presence of that precious idealised mother. We are told that these unconscious remnants of a still absolute passion for that mother (folle passion) survived from a happy period during the first years of life. His patients did not permit an easy access to that innermost possession. Notwithstanding the differences, I could say the same about my male patients in relation to their father (leaving aside for the moment their relationship to the original mother). To allow access to, and gradually to give up, this ideal father proved to be a most difficult and painful task. They surrendered it only after a strenuous and depressing battle of protest, as if desperately defending the last bastion in a besieged fortress.

In my conception of the mental structure of the mind, the ideal father is an essential ingredient of the ideal ego (idealised). By ideal ego I mean something different from Green's conception which he intimately relates to the 'purified pleasure ego'. I rather see the ideal ego as a minimally structured mental formation, belonging to the most archaic level of the mental representation of the self. It is related to the Ego ideal as the unconscious omnipotent fantasies are related to the more realisable and reasonable ambitions. The ideal ego is never directly affected by the superego. Unwittingly, my male patients retained the ideal father as a source of self-perfection through magical identification and for the sake of omnipotent, grandiose fantasies. They were also unaware of an implacable need to ensure that the analyst is and will remain a personification of that idealised figure. In order to keep things this way in the transference, these patients had to consolidate their actual identification with the failing father.

This determined resistance to the analytical breakdown of this neurotic equilibrium is related to the deep insecurity triggered by the exposure of the hidden ideal father. The patients much preferred to cling to the familiar than to trust the prospect of a change of object. The ideal father had to be unconsciously protected against time and change for the same reasons that applied in the case of the real father. Reality destroyed the idealised father and the unconscious phantasy wasted no time engraving deeply and permanently the image of the pre-traumatic father.

These analyses revealed that the panic anxiety experienced at the prospect of change arises from the belief that the threat of losing the first idealised paternal object involves the loss of one's own omnipotent feeling. The patients' self-esteem could not part with it, for the loss of omnipotence and invulnerability is felt as an experience of emptiness, of falling into the abyss, the loss of one's own self. These men were terrified by the perspective of becoming just ordinary people. They much preferred to remain dependent little boys, waiting.

An analogy could be drawn with the fetishist, without suggesting in the least that the ideal figure is a fetish. We know that the fetishist cannot accept that the woman has no penis because it would signify to him his own castration. Similarly, my patients cannot part with their ideal father because it would mean losing an essential part of their own mental constitution, with all the ensuing frightening feeling of emptiness involved.

Fluctuations in the transference

The deep-seated anxiety gave rise to a constant fluctuation of transferential psychological positions. Whenever the patients came close to overcoming their passivity and dependency, open rage and bitterness emerged. The analyst was then told that he was day-dreaming, harbouring an illusion, if he thought that a change was taking place. 'You thought you had been successful with me but your victory has been of short duration …'; or else: 'I have some news for you, I became passive again during the weekend … Without your presence I was unable to work … That is my true self … I am sorry to disappoint you …' All this is said with sarcasm, bitterness and almost with pride, barely concealing a feeling of triumph. They made it clear that they would go on forcing the analyst to father them. The narcissism had been transferred over to revolt, to passivity and to control over the object. These episodes revealed another paradox: while, on the more superficial (though unconscious) level they were compelling the analyst-father to remain the good and ideal father, at a deeper level they were proving him to be a failure by his inability to bring about any change in them. This represents one aspect of the secret, underlying, feeling of omnipotence.

On many other occasions we encountered in the transference another side of the same multi-faceted conflict. The introjected – and identified with – failing father was easily projected onto the analyst and the patient resumed once again the position of the bitterly disappointed little boy. The reproaches were numerous but one-sided: the analyst did not talk enough, did not interpret enough, did not support and encourage enough, did not participate enough; he refused to give advice and remained too distant, too uninvolved; he left the patient fatherless. These negative outbursts alternated with episodes of idealisation of the analyst, during which the patient found anew the justification to hold on to his passive dependency. The little boy was then happy, he had not lost his pride in his father. I repeat that this implies an ultimate paradox because, behind the syndrome of the happy little boy lies, deeply repressed, the scorn at the failing father; by remaining a little boy, the patient ensures that the analyst fails in his attempt to help him grow up.

Most of the time, these patients oscillated between two solutions: to remain the happy little boy recovering the ideal father or to resume the identification with the defeated castrated father.

The crushing primal scene

The second reason for avoiding change in the inner distribution of objects stems directly from the effect of the primal scene. When the analytical work finally undermined both the position of the ideal father and of the little boy, the patients felt called upon to assume the position of adult men, to assume a paternal function. This brought about a panic reaction: their unconscious knowledge reminded them that this meant being submitted to the same fate as their father, namely to be castrated and destroyed by the powerful mother – the powerfully destructive phallic mother. These patients have no ambiguity or doubt as to the final outcome of the primal scene: the mother destroys the father.

Not once did the opposite appear. During the phases of the analysis where the primal scene imagery was reawakened the patients, who happened to have previously recovered their sexual potency, lost it again; in no way could they dare penetrate a woman. At the risk of uttering a gross exaggeration, I would say that these men spent their life, after the trauma, in phobic avoidance of the dread of the primal scene. By so doing, the ideal father is spared the awful fate because he belongs for eternity to the pre-sexual time, the pre-Oedipal time. These patients harbour two major sources of anger: anger at the father for having let himself be destroyed by the mother, and at the mother for being ultimately destructive. It is only with my fetishist patients (males) that I have observed such a devastating internal action of the primal scene. The ideal father belongs to another world.

André Green reported that the complex of the dead mother led to a dramatic Oedipal phase. As the above remarks attest, it is clear that I have found the same with my male patients through the joint workings of the psychological loss of the father and the gloomy primal scene.

References

Abraham, N. and Torok, M. (1976) *The Wolf Man's Magic Word: A Cryptonymy*. Theory and History of Literature, vol. 37, Minneapolis: University of Minnesota Press, 1986.

Freud, S. (1917 [1915]) Mourning and melancholia. *S. E.* 14.

Green, A. (1983) *Narcissisme de vie, narcissisme de mort*. Paris: Editions de Minuit.

—— (1990) *La folie privée. Psychanalyse des cas limites*. Paris: Gallimard.

—— (1993) *Le travail du négatif*. Paris: Minuit.

—— (1994). *Un psychanalyste engagé. Conversation avec Manuel Macías*. Paris: Calman-Levy.

8

TAKING AIMS

André Green and the pragmatics of passion

Adam Phillips

What does the analyst want for the patient that the patient can, at least hope for, from the analyst? One of the striking things about André Green's writing has been his willingness to formulate answers to this question. Green has never been shy about making claims for analysis, about what psychoanalysis really is − both what it entails and where it cannot suspend its judgement − and thus what its aims might be. The idea of psychoanalysis as having aims (the relative freedom to love and work, the achievement of the depressive position, the capacity to play, the flourishing of one's true self) is one of the ways psychoanalysis makes sense of itself. An aim, after all, gives direction to our wishes, it gives hope a target. We think of the patient's purposes, his sense of direction, changing during an analysis, but not of the whole notion of a sense of direction being put into question. In psychoanalysis (both as theory and practice), the teleology of a life is recomposed but never disappears as a guiding principle. It gives the idea of the unconscious its necessary minimum of intelligibility: we may not know what we want, but we know that we want. We are always going somewhere for something.

Despite, or perhaps because of the rigour of his theorising − his always acute and incisive Freudian inductions − Green's stated aims of analysis have always been poignantly simple, with none of the covert moralism of the more esoteric versions of psychoanalysis.

Green writes:

> ...my hope at the end of the analysis will be, according to Freud's guidelines, that my analysand will be able to enjoy life a little more than he used to do before coming into treatment or, as Winnicott says, that he will be more alive, even if his symptoms do not all disappear.
>
> (Green, 1995b, p. 880)

163

And after going from Freud to Winnicott he can, as ever, make good his return to Freud: 'Is our psychoanalytic Puritanism,' he continues, 'responsible for the fact that we would consider sexuality as negligible in such enjoyment?' (Green, 1995b, p. 880).

Green says in an interview:

> What I think we are doing in analysis is to enable the people who come to us to increase their feeling of freedom. In what way? In order to liberate the forces which are present in themselves to enjoy life, not as scared people looking for all sorts of safety, nor as repenting sinners, but as human beings who are inhibited by something which makes them move on in quest of something they value. Analysis should improve their capacity to cathect something. We don't have to say what, they will find out ... In other words analysis should improve what the patient already has, or give him the possibility of finding that life is worth living.
>
> (Green, 1995, p. 25)

Enjoyment, aliveness, love of life, the feeling of freedom, cathexis as the quest for something of personal value, the possibility of what Green calls 'sexual ecstasy' (Green, 1995a); these, quite explicitly, are Green's values; the demands, one might say, he makes on analysis.

And yet, inextricable from these particular aims and inspirations, there is always another aim functioning ambiguously in Green's writing, as both a means and an end. 'Just as the instincts "seek representation", psychoanalysis can have no other aim than the working out of the activity of representation in the widest possible sense' (Green, 1991). 'So what should the aim of psychoanalytic work be?', Green asks elsewhere, 'To help the patient go as far as possible in the representation of his internal world and of his relationship to the external world as well, but mainly of the internal' (ibid.). In practical terms it is 'for the analyst to devote himself to the task of elaboration ... to give effect, albeit provisionally, to symbolisation which is always begun and never finished' (Green, 1983, p. 46). So for Green the 'only aim, in varying the elasticity of the analytic setting' (that is, in any way modifying the prescriptions of so-called classical analysis) is 'in searching for and preserving the minimum conditions for symbolisation' (ibid., p. 49). And because it is representation (the apparently fundamental capacity for symbolisation) that is, as it were, the aim and the object of analytic practice – then, what is the connection, if any, between what Green calls 'maximal symbolisation' and love of life? If, as Green suggests in a resonant sentence in his book on tragedy, 'The confusion between the unrepresentable and the non-represented seems to be the source of errors of interpretation' (Green, 1979, p. 30), then how would clarifying this confusion, if such a thing were possible, enable us to enjoy life a little more? Does maximal symbolisation (the hitherto unrepresented that is available for representation) lead to love of life – guarantee it, as it were? It is an act of faith (an act of Eros perhaps?) to believe that what is there to be represented, what can be represented, is necessarily on the side of a person's life. Green's work, in other words, circles around a question that seems almost quaint now: what kind of good can it do us to make the unconscious conscious? In what sense is loving (and therefore fostering) a representation of loving life? The belief that symbolisation is good for us (as a general principle, not, say, true for some people but not for others) is one of the foundational assumptions of psychoanalytic practice.

It is as difficult to define representation as it is to imagine an alternative to it. If, as Freud says in the phrase quoted by Green, that the instincts 'seek representation', it seems as if there is at least something (call it instinctual life, or even affect) to set against representation; something that is not yet in representational form. Words, like instincts, drives, urges, affects are, paradoxically our representations for whatever both seeks and resists representation. There is a story here about how something that is not language is turned into language; how the infant, or the body, articulates itself, engages in what Green calls 'the work of inner transformation'. Dreams and affect, and states of emptiness or absence have been the essential perplexities of Green's work because they are the areas of experience (or anti-experience) in which the nature of representation itself is put at risk: its very possibility is put in question. Representation is the individual's acknowledgement of insufficiency, his attempt to make more life rather than more death-in-life out of the inevitable (if temporary) absence of what he depends on. It is as though absence can only be borne if it is recognised as such: symbolisation, or the abolition of need. Green remarks:

> The dream remains a paradigm because it is the model for the whole of our work … the importance of the dream is closely linked to the importance of the concept of representation because, once again, what I think is most important is the dream representation, the thing which repeats itself in the absence of the object … the mind has the capacity to bring something back again which has been related to an object, without the object being there.
>
> (Green, 1979, p.30)

It is worth noticing here that Green does not say the object has been brought back, but something which has been related to an object, feeling for the object, desire for the object has been restored, via representation, in its absence. As though representation prevents our becoming oblivious of our affective life. 'In the end', he writes, 'what I maintain is that affect is representation', meaning that it can take no other form, or that affect in some way constitutes representation. 'Signifier of the flesh is what I proposed in Le Discours vivant. Today I would rather say the representative of passion'

(Green, 1980, p. 250). Analysis becomes a way of keeping our passions in play, 'the extension of the field of passion' (ibid.). The capacity for representation is deemed necessary (though not instrumental) to this project.

Our passionate selves are our best selves; and a passionate life is only possible, by definition, if we can make our passions known: to ourselves, by the absence of the object stimulating desire and its correlative representations, and to the object through the articulation of love as demand. There can be no passion – or rather, no recognisable passion – without representation. But this compelling psychoanalytic picture leaves us with a logical, and therefore an emotional conundrum: can there be passion without recognition? Is a private passion akin to the impossibility of a private language? Passion entails circulation and exchange; it is, in Green's felicitous phrase, a field. But why, after Green's uniquely interesting Freudian detour – after his own elaborations of Winnicott and Bion and his agonistic relation to Lacan – does Green end up with the traditional value of passion? What does his work add, or indeed does the relatively new work of psychoanalysis add to the old idea of passion; what further justifications does it offer?

'The object is the revealing agent of the instincts' (Green, 1991). More impressed by the immeasurable solitude of the baby than by its moments of contact – committed, that is to say, to primary narcissism rather than the consoling sociability of the newly over-observed infant (Green, 1995b) – Green has steered subtly between the Scylla and Charybdis of contemporary psychoanalytic theory. If we are endlessly offered either sexuality as the denial of the other (with its apotheosis in perversion) or concern for the other as denial of sexuality (with its apotheosis in reparation), Green nevertheless has been able to go on asking the Freudian question: what, if anything, has our passion got to do with so-called other people?

Green writes in his Sigmund Freud's Birthday Lecture,

> Again ... we are confronted with our ideology of what psychoanalysis is for. What is its aim? Overcoming our primitive anxieties, to repair our objects damaged by our sinful evil? To ensure the need for security? To pursue the norms of adaptation? Or to be able to feel alive and to cathect the many possibilities offered by the diversity of life, in spite of its inevitable disappointments, sources of unhappiness and loads of pain?
>
> (Green, 1995b)

Is passion – our anxious concern for the other – always, whatever else it may be, an idealisation of safety? Without a sophisticated capacity for symbolisation we can achieve none of the aims listed above, however ironically, by Green. In other words, there is nothing intrinsic in our capacities for symbolisation, that will make us more reckless: feeling alive is not bound up with our capacity for symbolisation, but with our use of that capacity.

Green's critique of psychoanalysis is only plausible because it implicitly acknowledges how representation can be the enemy of passion, and not merely when it is in the service of the death instinct. Kleinians promoting reparation, or ego-psychologists promoting adaptation both think of themselves as the guardians of Eros.

And yet, of course, to talk of the uses of representation – to talk pragmatically – in a psychoanalytic context, can only beg the question. In what sense, at least in psychoanalytic language, can we describe a person as choosing the use he will put his representations to? No one in the psychoanalytic community would claim to be speaking on behalf of the death instinct. And yet clearly one person's psychoanalytic aim (or ideal) can be another person's problem. It is curious how devoted one can be to the picture of a struggle (or indeed a war) between the life instinct and the death instinct – without there being any kind of consensus about how to recognise the workings of Eros. Reparation, adaptation, safety, aliveness, passion. Green, like anyone else, can assert his preference, but does it need backing from a god?

There is clearly a question here about how we go about legitimating our psychoanalytic aims, bound up as they are with fantasies about the kind of world we would prefer to live in. And this may not be a matter of providing foundations where none can be found, but rather of producing persuasive descriptions of why certain things, like aliveness or passion, might matter. How, if we take these things seriously, good things follow (if we start preferring aliveness, to adaptation, say, how will our lives be different?). If psychoanalysis saw itself as rhetoric rather than metaphysics (as persuading people to prefer certain ways of living to others, rather than revealing the truths about, and causes of themselves) we might have better descriptions not only of the aims of analysis, but of why we should value such aims. Slogans like 'Love and Work', for example, would be less likely to catch on so easily and we might be wondering then why so much of what Freud calls love sounds like work. So by way of conclusion I want to deduce, through a brief reading of Green's great paper, 'Passions and their vicissitudes', why it might be a good idea to value passion, and what Green adds to our common-sense view of passion that makes it even more attractive. It is one of the great virtues of Green's writing that it always performs what it claims to value: the work of transformation. One of the vicissitudes that the passions undergo in this paper is the imaginative work Green does on them.

For Green the question is not, is a passionate life a good life? but rather, given the passions, what life can we make that feels worth living? Passion, reduced to its scientific signifier, instinct, grounds the intelligibility, however vagrant, of both sanity and madness: 'instinctual life which is, after all, life itself' (Green, 1983, p. 244). As Green writes, passion is – whatever kind of mythological status we give it – the ultimate psychoanalytic referent. Without the life and death instincts, and their historical precursor, the passions, the human subject would seem disembodied. Now that the soul has fallen out of our vocabulary we are left with the passions as the heart of the mystery. It can only sound crass to talk of the pragmatics of passion (to ask why we might choose or value a passionate life over any other kind of life) because passion itself is *the* secular essentialism. The death of God can be proclaimed, but no one is going to celebrate the death of passion. As Green states quite explicitly:

> We know enough now to understand that passion, be it mad or psychotic, calls the tune ... [but] ... let us say to begin with that we (psychoanalysts) have taken care to recognise it only where it already exists. We have not introduced it. It is where it has always been. And if it was necessary to recognise it, it is because we undermined its importance.
>
> (1983, p. 241)

The paradox that Green begins with is that passion has always been there, but that psychoanalysis began with Freud trying to push it out of the picture, undermining it, as Green says (at least in translation), as though passion needed to be sabotaged. And now it needs to be reinstated, where it has always been. The return of passion as the repressed of psychoanalysis is the gist of Green's intent. This brings with it, of course, the assumption that something essential has been lost, and needs to be re-found.

For Green there is an 'original madness', not a psychotic core that defines the human subject and in his view Freud 'minimised ... the intrinsically mad essence' of the instincts. Original madness is no more and no less than the individual's inborn instinctual life. So to understand neurotic conflict, for example, as merely a question of superego prohibitions of the normal functions of nourishment, sexuality and work is consolingly bland. 'Should one not rather think that it is the risk of the appearance of this potential madness in the execution of these functions that makes it so dangerous to carry them out, and so implicitly disorganising for the ego' (ibid., p. 224). In other words, there is an excess here, an intensity of something, that psychoanalytic theory itself conspires to conceal. Freud failed with Dora, Green suggests, because he focused too much on her dreams, 'in other words, on her unconscious representations – while minimising her affects'; and because he was 'obliged to keep the transference outside the analysis, because with it the primacy of affects over representations appeared' (ibid., p. 225).

Representations, Green remarks, sustained a 'mediating distance' for Freud, ensuring he was 'well guarded against dangerous false connections'. There is something immediate, too present, too urgent, too invasive, called affect for which representation provides a boundary: both a barrier and a channel. But in the first act of the drama that is Green's paper there is, as it were, a natural antagonism between passion or affect and representation. And the 'dramatic' emblem of this antagonism is the sheer physicality of the hysterical fit, 'the element of passionate frenzy, linked to an instinctual upsurge' (Green, 1983, p. 221). There is an intensity of affect that representation cannot bind; the ordinary madness of love articulates, above all, the insufficiency of language. Passion without representation in autistic states or Green's blank psychosis is death-in-life, suicide by insulation; but the representation of passion ruptures language, reveals a daunting lack in representation itself. 'Fantasy binds libido to representations', Green writes; and yet,

> To concern oneself in preference to these representations is to analyse, but perhaps it is only to half analyse, if the suffering caused by this impossible love is not taken into account. It is to fix one's attention to the sexual theories of children while failing to recognise that the solution they present is only partial compared with the quantity of libido which they do not manage to bind by this means, and which remains a burden for the child.
>
> (ibid., p. 226)

Despite the technologies of technique (the elaborate sophistications of theory, the racket of profundity of competing analytic schools) psychoanalysis becomes simply and starkly: the emotional impact two people have on each other, whether they like it or not. 'It is a question', Green writes, spelling out the necessary impossibility of the venture, 'of binding an unquenchable libidinal tension through meaning' (ibid., p. 227).

Green's paper hurtles towards passion as catastrophe ('is passion the best or the worst of things? One is bound to admit that it is more often the worst than the best' (ibid., p. 236)) and towards the therapeutic pessimism that always follows in the wake of relinquishing all the versions of instrumental reason. Burdened by the burden of the child Green refers to, what is to be done? Is meaning, as it were, up to the task we have set it, or more often than not a betrayal masquerading as an affirmation, of the passionate life inside us? Having got himself into a familiar corner (and passion, after all is what always corners us), Green makes some useful distinctions in his defence of the very thing that leaves us defenceless. 'It seems to me essential,' he writes, 'to re-establish madness in the place where it has been recognised for all time: at the heart of human desire' (ibid., p. 239). And re-establishing it can only mean, given its rather obvious resilience, re-describing it in more promising form. If, as Green writes, 'Freud's logic is a logic of hope because it counts on wish fulfilment' (Green, 1980, p. 241), then passion is primordial hope.

Having shown the daunting incompatibility of representation and passion (and, of course, their necessary complicity – there can be no communicable, no hopeful passion without representation) Green describes how the mother is the one who gives the infant's passion a chance, as it were. His lucid distinction between madness and psychosis, and his account of the origin of psychosis ('Psychosis emerges when the subject is forced to mobilise his destructive instincts as a means to putting an end to a fusional relationship with a primordial object' (Green, 1983, p. 243)) are committed to the necessary value of binding the unbindable. 'Without representation instinct has become blind' (ibid., p. 240), he writes; but with representation what does it become? *Tolerable* is Green's word. Without representation the ego is overwhelmed, 'subject to the anxiety of separation and intrusion' (ibid., p. 246). And yet there is an equivocation here, an ambivalence about represen-tation that echoes throughout Green's work: the very thing that makes the individual's passion viable – representation – also gives it the lie. That representation is never good enough, and by the same token it is the only thing that is good enough.

Green leaves us with a contradiction that we should prefer to see as a paradox. On the one hand, he writes, 'I do not believe that affect escapes from symbolisation, or from metaphor' (ibid., p. 251); in other words, there is a sense in which affect can only reside in, be recognised through, its representations. On the other hand, implying as he has done throughout, that we may be bewitched (defensively over-impressed) by representations, he suggests in another personal confession: 'It seems to me that the attention given to representation comes from the concern for scientific demonstrability' (ibid., p. 250). And what then, we might wonder, is that a concern for? Cultural prestige, legitimation, reassuring forms of consensus? When Green, who has written with such illumination and consistency about negation writes, by way of internal debate, 'I am not saying that the work (in psychoanalysis) on representation is of little value ...' (ibid., p. 249), he gives us pause for thought. What else could we write about, or with, but representation? What would psychoanalytic practice be like, what would we do differently if (to reverse Green's earlier formula) we gave primacy to affect over representation? What Green's extraordinary Freudian meditation on passion leaves us with then is not the virtually nonsensical question: is keeping faith with representation keeping faith with passion? but the more pragmatic question, apparently incompatible with what we might think of as a psychoanalytic ethos, what kind of representations sustain our love of life, or foster that form of hopeful passion that Winnicott called aliveness, and that Green himself promotes? If we take seriously Green's preference for the Freudian language of pleasure and unpleasure, as opposed to the Kleinian language of good and bad, we would talk about a person's capacity or appetite for pleasurable forms of representation.

We need to distinguish, to tell the difference between what Green calls in this paper 'Freud's double equation, Eros = binding; destructive instincts = unbinding' (ibid., p. 248). This, of course, is the distinction that grounds all of Green's formulations and makes Bion's work integral to his own perspective. So it is instructive when, under the guise of being rather fussily punctilious, Green appears to under-emphasise a crucial point. He writes:

For binding and unbinding are always at work in madness as in psychosis. It is the resultant that counts, making transformations of the products of creation, or debris, products of disintegration. One must also insist, if one wishes to dot one's i's, on the positive role of unbinding, which produces discontinuity without which the mechanisms of recombination could not take place ....

(ibid., p. 249)

If there is a 'positive role' of unbinding, what are the criteria by which we recognise it? If unbinding makes possible a more fruitful binding, then Eros and the destructive instincts are collaborators and not exclusively antagonists. The individual's destructiveness may be integral, indeed essential to his passionate life, even if the consequent work of transformation seems to work against him. The logic of a life may be in excess of the distinctions we can make about it. Or, to put it another way, how does one know when someone is being self-destructive? To think of oneself as one's own best enemy implies an omniscient knowledge of what is good for one. Passion, as Green eloquently reiterates throughout this paper, leads people to apparently ruin their lives — 'acts which can compromise an entire life' (ibid., 1983, p. 222) — and yet from which of the many points of view in oneself is it ruin? 'Beyond the wish to recover', Freud says, 'the analysand clings to his illness'; Green writes, 'and I say that he prefers the object of his passion' (ibid., p. 251). A good life may entail the destruction of all that one apparently values; this is what Green intimates, this is the loophole he adds to our story of the passions. Passion always makes action morally equivocal. The passionate life is a good life because its goodness is always in question. Passion, Green stresses, is the object of analysis and sets the limit to analysability. It both tests and constitutes our capacity for representation; because it is a threat to this capacity, it is the source of its renovation. The life-line that is a death-line.

If 'The dead mother', whatever else it is, is Green's history of the psychoanalytic movement — a history of analysts brought up by, trained by, analysts mourning the death of the analytic parents — then 'Passion and its vicissitudes' is Green's *Genealogy of Morals*. Green's psychoanalytic aims, after all, cannot help but echo Nietzsche's paradoxical moral aim of 'more life'. And the dead mother, in Green's description, turns the infant's passions to persecutions. It is the fate of the analyst's passions — in the practice of analysis, bound and unbound by the analytic setting — that provides the sub-plot, the uncomic relief, of these remarkable twinned papers. How does the analyst keep his love for analysis, his aliveness to the work? The passion for analysis, one might say, is the struggle against the dead mother. But if the passion for analysis is merely the analysis of passion, then what is the analyst consigning himself to?

References

Green, A. (1979) *The Tragic Effect*. Cambridge: Cambridge University Press.

—— (1980) Passions and their vicissitudes. In A. Green *On Private Madness*. London: Hogarth Press and the Institute of Psycho-analysis, 1986.

—— (1983) The dead mother. In A. Green *On Private Madness*. London: Hogarth Press and the Institute of Psycho-analysis, 1986.

—— (1991) Instinct in the late works of Freud. In *On Freud's 'Analysis Terminable and Interminable'*, edited by Joseph Sandler, New Haven: Yale University Press, 1991, 124–41.

—— (1995a) An interview with André Green. *New Formations* 26: 15–35.

—— (1995b) Has sexuality anything to do with psychoanalysis? *International Journal of Psycho-Analysis* 76: 871–83.

9

THE INTERPLAY OF IDENTIFICATIONS

Violence, hysteria and the repudiation of femininity

Rosine Jozef Perelberg

Introduction

André Green is one of the most important contemporary psychoanalysts to have followed the line of enquiry Freud inaugurated from the 1920s onwards, when he confronted the limits of psychoanalysis through the elaboration of the concepts of the death instinct, primary masochism and the repudiation of femininity (Freud, 1920, 1924, 1937). Green has pursued his research into the work of the negative and the polysemic dimensions it may take (1993), and has been concerned to understand the phenomena which are potentially at the limits of symbolic representation, not only due to mechanisms of repression, splitting, denial and negation, but also because they relate at the same time to something profoundly destructive in the psychic sphere that breaks through the capacity of the mind to contain it. Green has been interested in the 'death-like quietus out of emptiness and nothingness' (1980, p. 55), which he has identified in his work on clinical expressions of the negative: 'The category of "blankness" – negative hallucination, blank psychosis, blank mourning, all of which are connected ... with the problem of emptiness, or of the negative, in our clinical practice.' They are, Green suggests, 'the result of one of the components of primary repression: massive decathexis, both radical and temporary, which leaves traces in the unconscious in the form of "psychical holes" ' (1980, p. 146).

André Green has played a leading role in pushing psychoanalytic enquiry into the areas of borderline states and psychosis: 'this is where the future of our work lies' (personal communication). In turn, developments in the understanding of borderline states in the last twenty years may shed further light into some points already delineated at the time 'The dead mother' was published. The themes presented in this seminal paper constitute not only general features of the borderline patient's system of internal object

173

representations (or, of course, such patients' lack of such a stable system), but, following the tradition of Freud and later Winnicott, emphasise the relevance of the loss of the object for the structuring of the mind. The themes that underlie the 'dead mother' configuration refer to a specific state of mind, and not necessarily to an actual state of the mother herself. Green emphasises that the dead mother is 'a revelation of the transference' (1980, p. 148). I suggest that the concept might be regarded as a 'core complex' in borderline states, equivalent, perhaps to Glasser's core complex in perversions (1979).

In this chapter I would like to explore the way in which Green's ideas on the negative have inspired my understanding of two main types of psycho-pathology: violence and hysteria. I would like to suggest that what lies at the basis of violence (in some patients) and hysteria is the repudiation of femininity. While hysteria takes the person's own body as the vehicle for the expression of the drama of the conflict between identifications, in violence there is an externalisation of the drama. In both, the 'drama' seems to me to be secondary to the primary conflict. Green has suggested that: 'Manifestations of hatred and the following process of reparation are manifestations which are secondary to this central decathexis of the maternal primary object' (1980, p. 146). Both symptomatologies point to the limits of what can be expressed through representations. 'A feeling of captivity ... dispossesses the ego of itself and alienates it to an unrepresentable figure' (ibid., p. 153). Green suggests a crucial point of technique: 'to interpret hatred in structures which take on depressive characteristics amounts to never approaching the primary core of this constellation' (ibid., p. 146).

In this chapter I will discuss violence with reference to a male patient who has been in analysis with me for many years.[1] My thinking about hysteria will just be outlined and will centre on some thoughts about Anna O, the result of research I was able to embark on recently.[2] I would like to suggest that both violence and hysteria may be understood as attempts by the individual, overwhelmed by the fluidity of their identificatory processes to repudiate their feminine, passive, identification. My patient's feminine identification is ultimately given representation in a dream, in the sixth year of analysis, of being buried inside a coffin in a state of sedation; Anna O's hysteria was expressed through an experience of void, paralysis, lapse of memory and abolition of time: white, empty, blank, categories that André Green has developed.

Identification as a mode of thinking

In his letter of May 1897 to Fliess, Freud described identification as *a mode of thinking* about objects (Masson, 1985). This mode of thinking lies at the origin of the constitution of the individual, through a series of modifications of the ego. It is an *unconscious* process that takes place in *phantasy*. In the early modalities of identification, mental processes are experienced in bodily terms such as ingesting or devouring. It is through the process of internalisation and the progressive modification of the ego, through the differentiation between ego, superego and id – each ruled by different timings – that the individual is constituted. These identifications, by definition unconscious, are in conflict with a sense of 'I' as the centre of the subject and this is one of the several revolutions introduced by psychoanalysis in terms of its thinking about the individual. The individual is not the 'I'. In the poet Rimbaud's formula: 'I am another' (in Lacan, 1978, p. 17). The individual in psychoanalytic thinking is thus engaged in a process of *exchange* with the other.

Identification, as a mode of thinking, presupposes a fluidity between different positions and ideas, and is present in all individuals. Freud's fundamental views about sexuality throughout his work concerns the fluidity between masculinity and femininity:

> psychoanalysis cannot elucidate the intrinsic nature of what in conventional or in biological phraseology is termed 'masculine' and 'feminine': it simply takes over these two concepts and makes them the foundation of its work. When we attempt to reduce them further, we find masculinity vanishing into activity and femininity into passivity, and that does not tell us enough.
>
> (Freud, 1920:171)

In this chapter I discuss the interplay between 'identification' and 'identity', the 'individual' and the 'person' and suggest some implications they have brought to the understanding of material derived from my clinical practice in the following ways (Perelberg, 1997, 1998).

First, I have come to understand that *in certain individuals the fluidity of identificatory processes becomes overwhelming for the mind, because of the lack of distinction between phantasy and reality.* Such fluctuation is indeed common in borderline patients. I think that some violent patients attempt to immobilise a specific aspect of the whole range of identificatory attributes in order to establish a *persona*, an *identity*.

Second, I further suggest that *violent behaviour may be an attempt to prevent the extreme fluidity between masculine and feminine identificatory processes and avoid the recognition of a profound sense of entrapment inside a female figure.* The physical act of violence may be an attempt to create a mental space in relation to confusing internal primary objects, locked in a violent primal scene, particularly in relation to the mother.

Third, these ideas are to be understood in terms of the *narcissistic structures of the violent patient, who attempts to evade the experience of relating.* Green defines narcissism as fundamental resistance to analysis. 'Doesn't the defence of the One imply the refusal of the Unconscious just as the Unconscious implies the existence of a part of the psychic apparatus which has a life of its own, which defeats the empire of the ego?'.[3] This allows one to suggest that while most neurotic individuals may take their 'identity' for granted, it becomes a major issue for the borderline and narcissistic personalities.

Fourth, it is my understanding that *in the violent patient there seems to be a passage from an 'unconscious phantasy' to a 'delusional system' in response to a need to separate from internal objects through external violence.* If we accept Freud's formulation that phantasies of violence in the primal scene are universal, in some violent patients these phantasies seem to acquire the status of actual beliefs.

Fifth, if violence, for some patients, is an attempt to immobilise the experience of an extreme mobility of internal identificatory processes, I would then suggest that a technical challenge in the analysis of these patients is to identify and keep in mind the *shifts between the identificatory processes* and formulate them in terms of interpretations to the patients.

Finally I will try to indicate that as the analyst is progressively more able to identify the patient's internal movement between different states and identificatory processes and able to integrate these into interpretations to the patient, the patient is himself more able to tolerate the internal fluidity between identificatory processes.

I will now examine material from the five times a week analysis of a violent young man, which has been the source of some of these thoughts.

A case of violence: clinical material

The main information Karl brought up about himself at his first consultation was his special relationship to his mother. Karl is in his early twenties; his father left his mother when she was pregnant with him. His mother married when he was still a baby. Three years later the couple had a baby girl; and two years later they had another girl. Karl feels, however, that his mother always let him know that he was the most important person in the family for her. At the same time, he experiences his mother as unable to tolerate his sexuality or, even less, him being a man. His father was violent towards him throughout his childhood, hitting him frequently about the head. He recalls being frightened of his father. When he was 18, Karl decided to study martial arts; he feels that his father then became frightened of him and stopped hitting him.

The analytic process: the patterns of the transference

At his first consultation Karl presented me with a question that he felt had become an obsession for him and which expressed his concern about the nature of his parents' sexuality. He told me that his parents were involved in 'sado-masochistic games'. He had known this since childhood because he and his sister had listened to them behind their bedroom door. During this same consultation, Karl started to let me know about the extent of the violence in which he had been engaged. At university, he had become involved in serious violent situations with other young men (an example was that of a fight where he and other youths had used broken bottles and which had left him in hospital with 15 stitches in his head) and in escalating violence in his sexual relationship with a girlfriend. At that first consultation I noted the possible unconscious association between his question about the nature of his parents' sexuality and his own relationships with male and female friends.

In tracking the way in which Karl related to me in his analysis I progressively came to understand that each time his analyst understood him, he attempted to escape from an experience of having a mind. He then had to disappear by not coming to his sessions for a time. At the beginning of the analysis this was expressed basically in the states of sleep Karl would get into, from which he could not be awakened, neither by several alarm clocks nor by his mother shouting at him. He could disappear from the sessions for a week, for instance, without realising that so long had passed since his last session. The interpretations, during this period, consistently pointed to this complete retreat both from the encounter with the analyst and from the obstacles Karl inevitably experienced in his relationship with me. At this time, Karl's sleep was dreamless, and this was also interpreted as a flight not only from me, but also from the experience of having a mind. Karl also spent a great deal of time compulsively playing computer games where violence was expressed in a robotic way against dehumanised enemies.

Karl gradually revealed how difficult it was for him to maintain contact with real living people, since this involved levels of frustration, violence and terror that he simply could not tolerate. Yet, as his confidence in the analytic relationship grew, his thoughts and aggressive interactions outside the sessions became more vividly present in his accounts during the sessions. At times he inundated me with accounts of extremely violent behaviour which left me disgusted, frightened and hopeless about the possibility of my having any impact on him.

At this stage, I felt able to say no more than that his violence seemed to follow on from his fear of my intrusiveness in the transference. He responded by telling me that he possessed a gun and bullets, which he kept at home. As he talked about this, it seemed that he was keeping a part of both himself and myself hostage, terrorised by his potential destructiveness. At that point I seriously considered terminating his analysis.

Inevitably, my interpretations were rooted in my countertransference: he needed to know that he could terrify me as a way of protecting himself from his own fear of me.[4] My interpretations allowed him to get rid of the gun but this left him without the power to terrorise me; he felt lost, abandoned and deeply depressed. To counteract his depression, he intensified his accounts of criminal activities. After a period in his analysis in which I consistently interpreted to him the function of his criminal activities as a means of creating a distance from me and the analysis, he was able to understand and acknowledge that it was easier for him to come to the sessions after dangerous criminal encounters, such as obtaining and selling stolen diamonds, which gave him a sense of omnipotence. I also suggested that this was because he felt less frightened of my power over him. His criminal activities thus served to distance him from me and while they had many determinants, one transferential aspect was undoubtedly the wish to avoid a meaningful emotional relationship.

The alternation between presence and absence, life and death, love and hate

At the beginning of his analysis Karl had many dreams that portrayed his experience of himself as inhuman, machine-like, deprived of feelings and thoughts. He dreamt that he was a computer or of being different kinds of monsters; in one particular instance he was a monster that was disintegrating. In the clinical material which follows one can identify a trajectory whereby Karl was able to bring to the analysis images that express his terror of losing himself and becoming imprisoned, and of being manipulated by a lethal couple. I will indicate a progression in his analysis to a capacity to experience himself in a more humane way.

At the beginning of the third year of analysis, though, the image Karl spoke about most frequently was that of a disembodied head that did not belong to him. This image was derived from a television play by Dennis Potter that had made a strong impression on him. In one particular session, Karl came in and threw himself on the couch. He started telling me about watching *Cold Lazarus* by Dennis Potter on TV. He said he was not sure what about the play had caught his attention so much. Thinking about it had prevented him from sleeping at night. It was something to do with the language. He had watched it on both Sunday and Monday and explained that the play was being shown on two channels. He told me the story, saying that it was science fiction and thus something to which he would immediately be attracted. In the story, a man has his brain cryogenically preserved in the hope that it could be revived many years later, 400 years into the future. In the play, the man's memory was being revived by two scientists. Karl said that it had been something in the quality of the language that had arrested his attention. It was like a language without a link with anything else, coming straight from the head. It reminded him of himself when his mental state was not good. The thing about this man was that he was just a head so that in a way his memories did not belong to him. *He did not have an identity.* He was just what this couple of scientists did with him.

I said that he was describing a quality he could identify in himself when he was avoiding having any feelings and was talking from his head only. He then said that when he was in that state of mind – without feelings – *he felt that he did not have an identity.* His identity had then been taken over by another part of him – the 'scientist' – who he felt was in control. He said that there was a connection between that play and *Karaoke*, another play by Potter in which a character, who is an author, feels that people around him are repeating lines from his plays, which are being fed back to him about his own life. I then spoke to Karl about his experience of relating to other people: he too feels that he can only re-find his own lines. Later in the session, I pointed out that there was also the issue of possession: is he a possession of mine or am I a possession of his?; there is no one who can have a life of their own, a 'real identity' (his term). Violence becomes Karl's solution to this dilemma.

Karl then told me about a dream: *there were three men, a weak man, a bodyguard and a violent man, who was able to overcome the bodyguard.* In his associations Karl spoke of 'great men', such as Rabin or Kennedy, who were nevertheless in a fragile position. We understood this dream as expressing the various experiences he had of himself. Underneath the bodyguard there was a fragile man, who was afraid of being hit by the violent aspect of himself.

A more three-dimensional experience of himself had, however, started to emerge in his analysis, as we also identified that it was the bodyguard – the man 'in between' – who tended to come to the sessions. Karl was, however, afraid of being left with a perception of himself as a weak and unprotected man who was bound to get killed. In the transference I was at the time acutely aware that I needed to keep all three aspects of him in mind.[5]

However, there was also an emphasis on the inevitability of death, as I could not avoid pointing out at the time. Karl then disappeared from a few sessions and when he came back he brought another dream: *Karl was inside a tomb and a panther was approaching him. He was terrified as the panther came closer and closer, and he woke up terrified.* In his associations, Karl remembered first seeing a panther during a trip to the West Indies with his mother, who had taken him on a visit to a friend who kept a panther as a pet. In the session, we were able to understand that the tomb was where he felt he had been for the week he had been absent from the sessions, and that he was now afraid of me, a panther, which posed a danger to him as representative of the outside world. He was, however, also afraid that, like his mother's friend and his own mother, I would want to keep the panther in him as my pet.

This opened up his memory of a film called *The Vanishing*, which he told me was the most terrifying film he had ever seen in his life. In the film, a man called Hoffman had lost his girlfriend. She had vanished in a petrol station and he had spent three years looking for her. Throughout this period, he kept getting letters from a man saying that he had made her disappear. This man tortured Hoffman in this way for three years; when they finally met, he told him that he, Hoffman, could take him to the police if he wanted, because there were no traces whatsoever of what he had done. The only way Hoffman could find out what had happened to his girlfriend was to go through the same thing as her. Hoffman thought long and hard; in the end he decided that he had to find out what had happened. He took the tranquilliser this man gave him, and at that moment he was sealing his fate. He fell asleep and woke up in a coffin, buried under the earth. It was the most terrifying experience anyone could think of, to be buried alive.

He then said that a scene that he could not forget took place in a car, when Hoffman became friendly with the fascist psychopathic kidnapper. Hoffman laughed with him and said that all his life he had done what was expected of him. He said that one knows that people who are kidnapped sometimes become friends with their kidnappers, like people who are kidnapped by Arabs and then come back to the West mad, holding the Koran and claiming that their kidnappers are in fact good people. Karl told me about an American version of the same story made by the same director, with Jeff Bridges in the leading role, which had been a disaster. They had changed the ending so that Hoffman is saved by (Karl laughed) 'John Wayne'. Later Karl added that in fact it had been this man's girlfriend who saved him just as he was being buried.

I said to him: You know I think that it was terrifying for you to see in this film the way you bury yourself alive in your bed/coffin. You are terrified of experiencing yourself either like Hoffman, who takes the tranquilliser, or the psychopath/murderer who gets a kick out of it and out of having killed the girlfriend three years ago (the analysis). I also feel, however, that it is terrifying for you to wake up and find yourself in the coffin. (Equally, I thought that he was also terrified that trusting me was like taking the sedative that would lead him to feel buried in my couch and thus converted to the Koran, my mad version of things.) He was very struck by all this. He said that he could understand what I was saying but he was not really afraid of me now. I added something about his misgivings about the ending. He thought that the version of the movie with a happy ending had been a disaster, in contrast to the terrifying one. He had also pointed out the fact that it was the man's girlfriend who had saved him, not John Wayne. I felt that this showed his mixed feelings about the idea of a girlfriend/woman analyst saving him.

I thought this session was important. Karl had himself found a narrative and an image that referred to his own experience of his two states – being dead and the terrifying waking up: the wish to be 'saved' but also the terror of being saved by another entrapping/dead/not birth-giving woman/mother/analyst, ultimately the fear of a couple made up of the murderer and the coffin, a couple which was not life-giving and which, ultimately, lived inside him. What I felt was so important in this session was the way in which we were able to identify these various positions within himself: the murderous couple and the victim who was being murdered.

Karl missed the next session and on Friday he said that he had been unable to wake up on Thursday. He could not understand why. He talked about his relationship with his girlfriend, the first real relationship in his life, which he felt had changed him. Then he talked about a film called *A Matter of Life and Death* which was one of the most beautiful films he had seen. David Niven plays a pilot in the Air Force during the war whose plane has been attacked. He falls through the air and Death comes to fetch him. It is, however, very foggy, so Death cannot find him. In the meantime, a woman hears David Niven on the radio when he is hit and she falls in love with him. She goes to find him in the hospital and they fall in love. Then Death catches up with him and the rest of the film is about the trial at which David Niven defends himself. He says that because of these two days, he has fallen in love, that it is not his fault they missed him, but now he needs his life extended. The judge has the power to decide whether to extend his life or not. In the end the judge decides to let him live. It was really a most striking film, Karl added. The title was most appropriate, truly 'a matter of life and death'.

I said that he felt that his analysis and his analyst had changed the course of his life, but that this put him, at the same time, in the hands of a judge who has to decide whether or not he can carry on living (or having his analysis). He is not sure if the judge is going to be benign or not. Karl said that he was not used to meeting benign people in his life. I pointed out the contrast between *A Matter of Life and Death* and *The Vanishing*, the former expressing the capacity for love, the latter the destructive/fascist forces inside him. I said that I thought it was difficult to find connections between these two films, these two experiences within himself. He was quiet for a moment (a rare experience). Later in the session I said: 'You know, I think that today you want me to know that there is a loving, devoted part of you as well.' He said that this session had been really amazing!

Discussion

Phantasy and beliefs

Britton has proposed a distinction between phantasy, belief and knowledge. He suggests that '*belief* is an ego activity which confers the status of psychic reality on to existing mental productions (phantasies)' (1995, pp. 19–20). I think these distinctions are useful in that for my patient, his unconscious phantasies about the primal scene have the status of beliefs. In Karl's thinking there is also a lack of differentiation between life and death and a terror of finding out that he is establishing an identity between the two.

While he is asleep in the coffin, Hoffman is not aware of his predicament, which I think includes the question of whether he is submitting to a man (Hoffman) or to a woman (or a woman's womb = the coffin). It is only when he wakes up that he is terrified by the fact that he is trapped inside the coffin, which can ultimately be experienced as the combination of a parental couple which is not life-giving: the psychopathic father who commits murder by burying him, and the entrapping mother who does not allow him to be born or to live outside her body and her mind. The coffin was also the couch, the 'bedrock' of his analysis and where he was afraid of waking up to

181

find out that he had submitted to a couple who had committed murder in the primal scene. In a state of ultimate sleep without any dreams, I think Karl attempted to remove all representations from his mind. The counterpart to that is the violence, where all this gains representation (as expressed in the derivatives of his unconscious phantasies in his analysis) and has to be expressed in action

Hysteria: the case of Anna O

Anna O has fired the imagination of many psychoanalysts and a great deal has been written about her.[6] I will provide only minimal information, in order to outline some of my thoughts.

Anna O started her 18-month-long treatment with Breuer, when she was 21 years old. Her parents had four children, three daughters (of whom she was the only survivor at the time she met Breuer) and a son, 18 months younger than her. She had been looking after her father who was ill with tuberculosis for some five months, doing the night shifts, while her mother looked after him during the day, when Breuer first saw her. Anna O initially started to suffer from coughing, sleepiness and agitation in the afternoons. After the beginning of the treatment with Breuer she developed a variety of other symptoms: ocular disturbances, paralyses, contractions, linguistic disorganisation (when she also spoke a mixture of five languages) and later mutism. She also had hallucinations of snakes. Once, while nursing her father, she had a hallucination of a black snake that was about to bite him. She tried to move her arm but was unable to do so, as it became paralysed. She tried to pray but could only remember the lines of an old English nursery song (Humpty Dumpty). She looked at the fingers and each had become a little black snake; each nail, a skull. After her father's death, four months later, Anna O suffered from a 'negative instinct', recognising no one in her household and speaking only in English to Breuer. She also developed different personalities, at different times: initially a good one and a naughty one, later; one who lived in the present and another who lived 365 days earlier. It has been reported that on the last day of her treatment with Breuer, Anna O displayed hysterical symptoms of a pregnancy, showing 'contractions' and saying: 'Here comes Dr Breuer's child'.

Anna O herself designated her treatment with Breuer as her 'talking cure' and referred to the cathartic method as 'chimney sweeping'. In 1953 Ernest Jones revealed the identity of Anna O. Her real name was Bertha Pappenheim, who, ten years after her treatment with Breuer had become an important social worker and feminist in the Jewish Community, saving the lives of many orphans from pogroms in Eastern Europe, and Jewish women who were being sold as slaves.

Hysteria, bisexuality and primal scene

Hysteria and bisexuality have an essential link for Freud, who suggested that hysterical attacks express an experience of rape in which the hysteric plays both roles. It is a question of shifting identifications in an attempt to retain one identification, which is phallic. This is also present in the violent patient. 'In one case I observed, for instance, the patient pressed her dress up against her body with one hand (as a woman), while she tried to tear it off with the other (as a man)' (Freud, 1908, p. 166).

It was in the discussion of the case of Katharina, that Freud himself first related hysteria to the primal scene (1893–95). Freud mentioned at least three further cases linking anxiety to the primal scene (in a letter to Fliess, in his paper on anxiety neurosis (1895), and in his analysis of Dora), although, throughout his work, he oscillated between regarding this as a 'real event' and a 'phantasy': 'I maintained years ago that the dyspnoea and palpitations that occur in hysteria and anxiety neurosis are only detached fragments of the act of copulation' (1905: 80).

In a later letter to Jung in 1909, Freud wrote about Anna O's term 'chimney sweeping': 'The reason why a chimney sweep is supposed to bring good luck is that sweeping a chimney is an unconscious symbol of coitus, which is something of which Breuer certainly never dreamed' (E. Freud, 1960, p. 161).

Freud attributed increasing importance to primal scene phantasies and later in his work he linked the origins of the function of phantasysing itself to these primal phantasies. According to him there is a specific, imaginary configuration to these primal scenes: they represent a scene of violence, where the father is inflicting pain on the mother (Laplanche and Pontalis, 1985). He later suggested that hysterical attacks represented phantasies about the sexual encounter as a scene of rape. In one of Bertha Pappenheim's plays, *Women's Rights*, the sexual act is represented as an aggressive act, a rape and surrender to the enemy. A woman was raped and impregnated by her lover, who was already married and who then left her.

Anna O's symptoms started at her father's bedside when he became ill. She started to cough when he was dying of tuberculosis, revealing her unmistakable identification with her father: when she looked at herself in the mirror it was his skull that she saw.[7] At his bedside, the fingers in the shape of skulls, which Britton convincingly suggests refer to masturbation, are a reminder of Freud's text 'A child is being beaten' according to which the wish to be loved by the father is transformed into the phantasy of 'a child is being beaten' (where the individual disappears from the scene) (1919). This central phantasy links masochism and femininity and expresses the guilt feelings for the incestuous desires towards the father. Breuer wrote in his 1882 report that Anna O had 'truly passionate love' for her father (Ellenberger, 1972, p. 267). Freud, however, also suggested that, at its core, hysteria indicates a relationship with a hated object.

In his analysis of melancholia, Freud showed that the ego can treat itself as an object and is able to direct against itself the hostility which relates to an object. He suggested that in melancholia 'the individual feels overwhelmed by guilt and hostility which become persecutory, demanding revenge and expiation' (1915, p. 252,). One could understand Anna O's symptoms as expressions of struggles with her melancholic state and as transformations of her mourning into sexual excitation (Braunschweig and Fain, 1975).[8]

The famous accounts of hysterical patients – Anna O, Lucy R, Elizabeth Von R, Dora – indicate that they have all been disappointed by their fathers – through illness, impotence, weakness and death. Coupled with this picture of disappointment with the father is the longing for another woman who becomes the personification of unattainable femininity, like Dora's longing for Mrs K. Is it that with the father's weakness, illness, impotence or death, the daughter becomes frightened of being at the mercy of an internal imago of the mother?

In the years between 1920 and 1925 a new dimension appears in Freud's writings in relation to his understanding of female sexuality. The daughter's love for her father covers a more fundamental and older love, related to the mother. In a letter to Stefan Zweig in 1932, Freud wrote about Breuer's flight from Anna O when he heard about her hysterical pregnancy: 'At this moment he held in his hand the key that would have opened the doors to the "Mothers", but he let it drop.' The reference to the 'Mothers' is an allusion to Faust's mysterious researches (in Goethe's *Faust*, Part II, Act I). Is this Freud's intuitive view of what Anna O's father's death left her grappling with, her unconscious feelings towards her *mother*? Breuer himself made this reference at the end of the first section of the theoretical chapter of his book. The mysterious mothers are goddesses who dwell below, in an internal *void, without space, place or time* (in Pollock, 1968). Are these not markedly similar to what Green describes as the expressions of the negative? Does this not, therefore, suggest a link between the negative and femininity?

It is interesting to link these ideas about the 'mothers' world to the episodes of depersonalisation, mutism, paralysis, 'time-missing' and gaps in memory that followed Anna O's hallucination of the snake. They are interruptions in the domain of a reality which is being disavowed, indicating perhaps what Britton has designated in his book as a 'suspension of belief' (1998, p. 15), when something is both known and not known at the same time. What is fundamentally known and not known is the fact of the division between the sexes (Freud, 1927; 1940; Chasseguet-Smirgel, 1964; Kohon, 1987). Sexuality is created through division and discontinuity (see Lacan, 1958; Mitchell, 1982; Rose, 1982), and these symptoms, paradoxically, seem to represent Anna O's identificatory struggles.

It is very striking that the literature on Anna O contains so little about her mother. It has been suggested that she had a negative relationship with her. We know that Anna O was between 9 and 10 months old when her mother became pregnant again and that this would have had an unconscious impact on her libidinal and aggressive investment in the primal scene (Freeman, 1972, and also Riccardo Steiner, personal communication). Breuer was oblivious to Anna O's reactions to his comings and goings and we do not know if these were experienced by Anna O as a repetition of earlier infantile experiences of abandonment by her mother.

At the onset of her father's serious illness Anna O lost her mother tongue and refused the nourishing environment representative of the mothering function which was taken over by Breuer. One could hypothesise that the erotic feelings towards a paternal analyst were defensive against both the risk of feeling paternal disappointment and of being left alone with a dangerous maternal introject. Through her rejection of her mother tongue, English became a language that she could share with Breuer, to the exclusion of everybody else. A phantasy of seduction indeed lies at the centre of Anna O's hysteria, and her treatment with Breuer indicates a confusion about who is the seducer.

If the hysteric is the feminine in the neurotic representation (Schaeffer), it is also the very repudiation of the feminine. Schaeffer (using an expression coined by Michel Cachoux) suggests: 'The Ruby is a stone that has a horror of red. It absorbs and retains all the other colours ... (but) rejects and expels red' (in Schaeffer, 1986, p. 925). Thus the hysteric has a horror of the colour red, of sexuality, while at the same time displaying it. In her hysterical pregnancy, paradoxically, Anna O was rejecting a feminine identification, the woman who would produce babies as a result of intercourse. This pregnancy may also be understood as her attempt to deny separation and to hold Breuer inside her, i.e. as a phantasy of incorporation. Denial and omnipotence constitute the first defences against the loss of the object, as Melanie Klein has suggested.

Some aspects of Bertha Pappenheim's later life represent transformations of Anna O's question, 'am I a man or a woman?' (See Leclaire, 1971; Kohon, 1984) albeit in a sublimated way. In her social work, she designated the social workers she trained as her daughters – products of an imaginary intercourse without a father or mother. The orphanage she built was known as 'Papahome', the house of the father, in which she would fulfil the two parental roles.

Hysteria becomes, fundamentally, a mode of thinking about sexuality and the sexual object (Schaeffer, 1986).[9] Hysteria works by imitation; the difference between identification and imitation is that between 'being like the object' and 'being the object'. Through her symptoms Anna O seems to be *imitating the sexual act. Her symptoms become like a theatre of the sexual act in an attempt to both deny and represent the primal scene and deny the mourning of her incestuous sexual desires.* It is also displaying a body that cannot be experienced as sexual and feminine but as bits and pieces that ache. The fracture of the mind (the Humpty Dumpty song she prayed at her father's bed) is mirrored in the fragmentation of the body through her symptoms.

Freud pointed out the fluidity which is the hallmark of identificatory processes. This fluidity contrasts with the individual quest for a *coherent* identity, a sense of cohesiveness that is denied him by the very nature of the psychic apparatus. It is, however, only the feelings of security engendered by attachments to objects of both sexes which prevent the individual from feeling overwhelmed by the pressure of the phantasies and desires, because they may then be anchored in a set of secure object relationships. Both Karl and Anna O might be seen as defending themselves against a wish for and terror of fusion with the dangerous mother. In Anna O's case, the mother seems to be absent through bereavement, maybe she is more like the 'dead mother' described by Green, although one needs to emphasise the speculative nature of these ideas, as we don't have access to the here and now of an analytic process that would allow the material to unfold in the transference. In Karl's case, the mother provides the experience of death – the coffin, ultimately, in the sense that she is not psychically able to give life. Is it that Anna O attacks in her own body the body of her mother, whereas Karl has to find in the other the (m)other?

Violence and hysteria may be seen as attempts to give birth to another person who is disconnected from the lethal parental couple and, *at the same time*, a repetition of the relationship attributed to this couple. Violence and hysteria may be seen as attempts to create personas detached from the conflict of identifications.

Issues of technique

In recent papers, Bateman draws on Rosenfeld's distinction between the two types of narcissism (1998, 1999), namely thick- and thin-skinned narcissists, and suggests that narcissistic and borderline patients tend to move between these two positions. Thin-skinned-narcissists are fragile and vulnerable, while thick-skinned narcissists are inaccessible and defensively aggressive. Bateman suggests that it is the movement between these positions that opens an opportunity for analytic treatment (1998).

I have found this suggestion extremely useful and would like to add in this chapter that it is extremely important that *the analyst is aware of this movement and takes it into account in their interpretations.* I think that Karl comes to his sessions at times when he is moving between positions – when he is the bodyguard in between the weak man and the killer, as expressed in his dream. However, as I came to realise, what characterises his movements in terms of their underlying phantasy is the alternation between an attempt to *retreat from a world of representations* (which he experiences as dangerous to himself as well as to others) on the one hand, to violence on the other. In other words a movement from a *blank space to violence*.

The blank space characterises his absences from the sessions, specially when he is locked in dreamless sleep, which I have come to understand ultimately as an attempt to create a space without obstacles, a space in which he identifies with an idealised mother in order to escape the terror of entrapment. In this state, Karl tries to deny access to any representation, both of the internal world (of phantasies), and of the external world (of thoughts, which require secondary process) in an attempt to reach a state of narcissistic closure. At the other pole, there is a massive entrance to the world of representation (in violence), which ceases to act as a representation and reaches the status of a belief. The alternation is thus between the blank space and the actual beliefs as expressed in violence. These two states may also reflect a massive split between an all-good world (blank) and an all-bad world that needs to be destroyed through violence. It is my suggestion that the analytic task becomes that of enabling the patient to be more aware of this alternation.

Green has pointed out an important technical dilemma in the analysis of the borderline patient in that analytic silence can be experienced as the silence of death:

> At one extreme is the technique proposed by Balint, which tries to organise experience as little as possible so as to allow it to develop under the benevolent protection of the analyst ... At the other extreme is Kleinian technique, whose aim is, on the contrary, to organise experience as much as possible through interpretative verbalisation.
>
> (Green, 1975, p. 56)

Green points out how – at the extremes – these techniques may correspond to the mother who is too absent, or the one who is too intrusive.

When Karl returned after missing many sessions (sometimes an entire week) he felt so excited about his achievement that it was as if a new life had started for him. He had survived whatever he felt he had been through. I came to realise that I had to keep in mind the *movement* between these two states, the presence and the absences, the sessions and the blank pages of the sessions he had missed. I had to keep in mind what he wanted to leave out, and attempt to capture the movement of the various identifications in between the sessions – and not just the temporary identity

I gradually understood that Karl was terrified by the link between these two states, a terror that left him confused and feeling without any control. My interpretations started to centre on this *link* between presence and absence, word and silence, masculine and feminine identifications, persecutor and persecuted, the written pages and the blank of the absences of the sessions. This took place progressively, in the verification of the pattern, and was given shape both in the dream about the tomb and in his response to the film *The Vanishing*: they were his representation of the world into which he had retreated and from which waking up was so terrifying. Karl has been more able to identify these oscillations himself, and has, for instance, linked not being able to come to sessions to something that he felt had frightened him in a specific session. I think he is less frightened of his oscillations between identifications and more able to talk about them.

Psychoanalysis is always characterised by an indeterminism, perhaps because phenomena are overdetermined so that many different phantasies are necessarily attached to the patient's symptomatology. The psychoanalytic task is consistently that of 'linking' affects, images and words as they are expressed and experienced in the transference and countertransference so that the preconscious may be constructed in this way.

The individual is thus placed in a chain of reciprocity in relation to his internal and external objects. I have previously suggested that Karl's fundamental concern in his analysis is to regulate his distance from his analyst (Perelberg, 1995). I can now understand this as representing his conflict about entering a chain of reciprocity that is, ultimately, the force of the life instinct itself. It has been Karl's inability to take part in this system of exchange that has condemned him to death itself, to his coffin. In his analysis we have been able to reach representations of this enclosure which, by definition, indicates his progressive entrance into the symbolic sphere.

© The Institute of Psycho-Analysis

Notes

1 This patient was seen as part of a subsidised scheme at the Anna Freud Centre in the Young Adults Research Group. This Research Group, whose clinical director is Mrs Anne-Marie Sandler, is composed of fifteen psychoanalysts who have undertaken analysis of young adults who suffered breakdown. I am grateful to the members of the group for helpful discussions of my patient. I am also grateful to André Green for his contribution when I presented a paper on this patient to the Paris Psychoanalytical Society in June 1998.

2 This was on the occasion of the 1998 English Speaking Conference, held in London, when I was the discussant of Ronald Britton's paper: 'Getting in on the act: the hysterical solution' (Britton, 1999). I am grateful to Riccardo Steiner for our conversations on Anna O.

3 'La défense de l'Un n'entraîne-t-elle pas *ipso facto* le refus de l'inconscient, puisque celui-ci implique l'existence d'une part du psychisme qui agit pour son propre compte, mettant en échec l'empire du Moi?' (1983, p. 9).

4 Being able to detect fear in me had the function of reassuring Karl that the fear was no longer in himself, so allowing him to feel safer. Sandler (1987) has suggested that in order to preserve its feelings of safety, the ego will make use of whatever techniques it has at its disposal. He gives examples of the way in which defence mechanisms can operate in the service of this 'safety principle'.

5 An important ingredient in Karl's analysis has been the accounts of films he has seen. At times, as in the sequence above, an account of a film, followed by an interpretation, was then followed by a dream. Money-Kyrle has suggested a theory of stages in representational thought that goes from a stage of concrete

representation (where no distinction is made between the representation and the object represented), through a stage of ideographic representation, as in dreams, to a stage of conscious and predominantly verbal thought (1968, p. 422). I think that for Karl films serve to contain projections of experiences before they can reach a stage of being able to be represented in dreams. The interpretations function as mediators in this process. This observation is in agreement with Sedlak's (1997) observation on the analyst's function in the transformation of patient's dilemmas into ones that can be thought and dreamt about, although in his paper Sedlak is addressing the role of the countertransference in the process.

6 In my PEP (Psychoanalytic Electronic Publishing) CD ROM search I was able to identify and visit 244 papers written on her between 1920–94. For the present chapter I have made use mainly of the following publications: Breuer and Freud (1893–1895), Ellenberger (1972, 1984); Freeman (1972); Peter Gay (1988) and Pollock (1968).

7 Britton has suggested:

> If I were to schematise Anna O's case ... I would see it beginning in the parental bedroom with her cough, starvation and progressive weakness; as a deadly union with a dying father; her cough was associated with dance music heard at the bedside and subsequently provoked by rhythmical music. The hallucination of the black snake then I take, to be death by intercourse and her death-head fingers a deadly form of masturbation. This was interrupted by her removal from the parental bedroom. Her subsequent paralysis expressed the infantile lack of locomotory power and the chaos of her movement and stiff-limbed contractures a caricature of a primal couple in intercourse. Her speech mirrored her limb movement; infantile, dislocated and polysyllabic.
>
> (Britton, 1999)

8 I think that mourning has an extreme importance in the understanding of the development of the transference and countertransference in Anna O's treatment with Breuer. Bertha Pappenheim's maternal grandmother had died when her mother was ten. Her mother had had three daughters of whom Bertha was the only survivor in 1881. Her sister Flora died at the age of two, four years before Bertha's birth, in 1859 (the same year that Freud was born). Her older sister Henrietta died of tuberculosis in 1867, at the age of 17, when Anna O was 8 years old. Wilhem, the only boy in the family, was born when Bertha was 18 months old. One can therefore imagine Bertha's mother as absorbed by bereavement as far back as her own childhood. Mourning had an important role for Breuer too: his mother, who had also been called Bertha, had died giving birth to his brother, Adolf, four years younger than himself. This brother died of tuberculosis at the age of 20. Breuer's own father died in 1872, when Breuer was 30 years old, eight years before he started treating Anna O. Breuer had himself five children, the older of whom, also called Bertha, was born in 1870.

9 Michel Fain has suggested that sexuality is a constant oscillation between hysteria and orgasm (in Schaeffer, 1986, p. 944).

References

Bateman, A. (1998) Thick- and thin-skinned organisations and enactment in borderline and narcissistic disorders. *International Journal of Psycho-Analysis*, 79: 13–25.

—— (1999) 'Narcissism and its relation to violence and suicide'. In R. J. Perelberg (ed.) *Psychoanalytic Perspectives on Violence and Suicide*. London: Routledge.

Bonaparte, M.; Freud, A. and Kris, E. (eds) (1954) *The origins of Psycho-Analysis: Letters to Wilhem Fliess, drafts and notes: 1887–1902*. London: Imago

Braunschweig, D. and Fain, M. (1975) *La nuit, le jour*. Paris: Presses Universitaires de France.

Breuer, J. and Freud, S. (1893–5) *Studies on Hysteria*. S. E. 2

Britton, R (1995) Psychic reality and unconscious belief. *International Journal of Psycho-Analysis* 76, pp. 19–23. Also in R. Britton (1998) *Belief and Imagination*. London: Routledge.

—— (1999) Getting in on the act: the hysterical solution. *International Journal of Psycho-Analysis*, 80: 1–14.

Chasseguet-Smirgel, J. (1964) Feminine guilt and the Oedipus complex. In Chasseguet-Smirgel, J. (ed.) (1985) *Female Sexuality*. London: Maresfield Gardens.

Ellenberger, H. F. (1972) The story of 'Anna O': a critical review with new data. *Journal of History and Behavioral Science* 8: 267–79.

—— (1984) Anna O: insight, hindsight and foresight. In Max Rosenbaum and M. Muroff (eds) *Anna O: 14 Contemporary Reinterpretations*. New York: The Free Press.

Freeman, L (1972) *The Story of Anna O*. Northvale, NJ: Jason Aronson.

Freud, E. L. (1960) *Letters of Sigmund Freud*, New York: Basic Books

Freud, S. (with Breuer, J.) (1893) On the psychical mechanism of hysterical phenomena: preliminary communication. S. E. 2.

—— (1895) On the grounds for detaching a particular syndrome from neurasthenia under the description 'anxiety neurosis'. S. E. 3.

—— (1905) Fragment of an analysis of a case of hysteria. S. E. 7.

—— (1908) Hysterical phantasies and their relation to bisexuality. S. E. 9.

—— (1909) Notes upon a case of obsessional neurosis. S. E. 10.

—— (1910) Leonardo Da Vinci and a memory of his childhood. S. E. 11.

—— (1911) Psycho-analytic notes on an autobiographical account of a case of paranoia (dementia paranoides). S. E. 12.

—— (1917 [1915]) Mourning and melancholia. S. E. 14.

—— (1919) 'A child is being beaten': a contribution to the study of the origin of sexual perversions. S. E. 17.

—— (1920) Beyond the pleasure principle. S. E. 18.

—— (1924) The economic problem of masochism. S. E. 19.

—— (1927) Fetishism. S. E. 21.

—— (1937) Analysis terminable and interminable. S. E. 23.

—— (1940) Splitting of the ego in the process of defence. S. E. 23.

—— (1960) *Letters of Sigmund Freud*. (ed. E. L. Freud). New York: Basic Books.

Gay, P. (1988) *Freud: A Life for Our Time*. London: J. M. Dent and Sons Ltd.

Glasser, M. (1979) Some aspects of the role of aggression in the perversions. In I. Rosen (ed.) *Sexual Deviation*. Oxford: Oxford University Press.

Green, A. (1968) Sur la mère phallique. *RFP*, 32(1): 1–38.

—— (1977) Atome de parenté et rélations oedipiennes. In C. Lévi-Strauss, *L'Identité*. Paris: Bernard Grasset (1977).

—— (1983) *Narcissisme de vie, narcissisme de mort*. Paris: Presses Universitaires de France.

—— (1975) The analyst, symbolisation and absence in the analytic setting. In A. Green *On Private Madness*. London: Hogarth Press (1986).

—— (1980) The dead mother. In A. Green, *On Private Madness*. London: Hogarth Press (1986).

—— (1993) *Le Travail du négatif*. Paris: Editions de Minuit.

Kohon, G. (1984) Reflections on Dora: the case of hysteria. In *International Journal of Psycho-Analysis* 65: 73. Also in G. Kohon (ed.) *The British School of Psychoanalysis: The Independent Tradition*. London: FAB, 1986.

—— (1987) Fetishism revisited. *International Journal of Psycho-Analysis* 68: 213–29. Also in G. Kohon (1999). *No Lost Certainties to be Recovered*. London: Karnac.

Lacan, J. (1978) *Le Séminaire, livre II. Le Moi dans la théorie de Freud et dans la technique de la psychanalyse*. Paris: Seuil.

——. (1958) *Le Séminaire, livre V. Les Formations de L'inconscient*. Paris: Seuil, 1998.

Laplanche, J. and Pontalis, J.-B. (1985) *The Language of Psychoanalysis*. London: Hogarth Press.

Leclaire, S. (1971) Jerome, or death in the life of the obsessional. In S. Schneiderman (ed.) *Returning to Freud: Clinical Psychoanalysis in the School of Lacan*. New Haven, CT, London: Yale University Press, 1980.

—— (1975) *On tue un enfant*. Paris: Seuil.

Lévi-Strauss, C. (1949/1969) *The Elementary Structures of Kinship and Marriage*. Boston: Beacon Press.

—— (ed.) (1977) *L'Identité*. Paris: Bernard Grasset.

Masson, J. M. (ed.) (1985) *The Complete Letters of Sigmund Freud to Wilhem Fliess, 1887–1904*. London and Cambridge, MA: The Belknap Press of Harvard University Press.

Mitchell, J. (1982) Introduction 1. In J. Mitchell and J. Rose (eds) *Feminine Sexuality – Jacques Lacan and the Ecole Freudienne*. London: Macmillan Press.

Money-Kyrle, R. (1968) Cognitive development. *International Journal of Psycho-Analysis* 49: . Also in D. Meltzer (ed.) (1978) *The Collected Papers of Roger Money-Kyrle*. Perthshire: Clunie Press, pp. 691–8.

Perelberg, R. J. (1981) Umbanda and psychoanalysis as different ways of interpreting mental illness. *British Journal of Medical Psychology* 53: 323–32.

—— (1995) A core phantasy in violence. In *International Journal of Psycho-Analysis* 76(6): 1215–31. Also in R. P. Perelberg (ed.) *Psychoanalytic Understanding of Violence and Suicide*. London: Routledge (1998).

—— (1997) Introduction 1. In J. Raphael-Leff and R. J. Perelberg (eds) *Female Experience: Three Generations of British Women Analysts on Work with Women*. London: Routledge (1997).

—— (ed.) (1998) *Psychoanalytic Understanding of Violence and Suicide*. London: Routledge.

—— (1999) The interplay between identifications and identity in the analysis of a violent man: issues of technique. *International Journal of Psycho-Analysis*, 80: 31–45.

Pollock, G. H. (1968) The possible significance of childhood object loss in the Josef Breuer–Bertha Pappenheim (Anna O)–Sigmund Freud relationship. *Journal of the American Psychoanalytic Association* 16: 711–39.

Rose, J. (1982) Introduction 2. In J. Mitchell and J. Rose (eds) *Feminine Sexuality: Jacques Lacan and the Ecole Freudienne*. London: Macmillan Press.

Rosenfeld, H. (1987) Afterthought: changing theories and changing techniques in psychoanalysis. In H. Rosenfeld *Impasse and Interpretation*. London: Tavistock.

Sandler, J. (1959) The background of safety. In J. Sandler *From Safety to Superego*. London: Karnac (1987).

Schaeffer, J. (1986) Le rubis a horreur du rouge. Relation et contre-investissement hystériques. In *Revue Française de Psychanalyse*, 50, May–June 1986, pp. 923–44.

Sedlak, V. (1997) The dream space and countertransference. *International Journal of Psycho-Analysis* 78(2); 295–305.

Wolleim, R. (1984) *The Thread of Life*. Cambridge: Cambridge University Press.

10

THE DYNAMICS OF THE HISTORY OF PSYCHOANALYSIS

Anna Freud, Leo Rangell and André Green

Martin S. Bergmann

In psychoanalysis some debates have acquired the status of landmark events, having determined the direction of the history of psychoanalysis. Among those I would count the debate on Ferenczi's active technique (1919–24) and the debate on Wilheim Reich's character analysis (1933) (see Bergmann and Hartman, 1976, parts 6 and 7). The Marienbad Symposium in 1936 seems also to belong to this category. There, for the first time, ego psychologists under the leadership of Otto Fenichel confronted the older generations of psychoanalysts. The best known of these debates, long kept secret but now available, are the controversial discussions between Melanie Klein and her circle, and Anna Freud and her followers (King and Steiner, 1991). To these well known examples, I suggest that we should add the London debate between Leo Rangell – supported by Anna Freud – and André Green, which took place in 1975.

The programme committee of the 29th Psychoanalytic Congress asked for two contrasting pre-published papers to serve as the basis for the plenary session, 'On Changes in Psychoanalytic Practice and Experience: Theoretical, Technical and Social Implications'. The psychoanalysts chosen were André Green and Leo Rangell. Anna Freud opened the discussion with her paper 'Changes in psychoanalytic practice and experience' (A. Freud, 1976). Shengold and McLaughlin summarised the debate. With the benefit of hindsight of over twenty years, I propose to examine the issues and what they can teach us about the dynamic forces that, largely unbeknownst to us, shape the history of psychoanalysis. Since these papers are easily available, my review will be brief, highlighting only what is significant for my purposes.

Rangell was asked to present the 'classical view' about changes in psycho-analysis. Of the three structures (superego, ego and id), the superego is, in Rangell's view, the most susceptible to outside influences. The id has probably not changed at all since the birth of psychoanalysis. The ego occupies an intermediary position between the two. He thought that

'Repression and the unconscious are permanent psychic attributes of men. What is repressed or what is allowed to escape repression changes before our very eyes, but the fact of repression remains unaltered' (Rangell, 1975, p. 90).

Rangell was willing to accept many changes provided they added, but did not substitute for the core of psychoanalysis. Additions should not be allowed to crowd out previous knowledge. The interpersonal and object relations schools should be rejected because they play down the role of the internal world. Self psychologists, who see the treatment of narcissism as a separate entity, are also mistaken. Narcissistic patients require no changes and no concessions in technique: 'The Oedipal phallic castration phase is a hub, a bull's-eye of psychoanalytic penetration, no area of the wheel of life is left out' (Rangell, 1975, p. 96).

Rangell's emphasis is on gradual peaceful evolution; no ominous clouds darken the horizon, no storm is expected, all is well with psychoanalysis. The rate of change in psychoanalysis should be kept to a minimum. What we have already acquired, we must preserve. I have shown elsewhere (Bergmann, 1998) that this optimistic attitude was characteristic of the Hartmann era. Ego psychology was initiated by Freud and elaborated by Anna Freud (1936) and Hartmann (1939), who attempted to put the ego on par with the id. In my monograph I have demonstrated that Fenichel was the leading ego psychologist before World War II. Fenichel did not value Hartmann's contribution highly; however, in the USA after World War II, Hartmann's monograph achieved canonical status. Rangell's presentation confronts us with an interesting historical problem. When does psychoanalysis develop in a slow and gradual way, as he wanted it to develop, and when do revolutionary changes take place? In retrospect, it seems that the publication of Loewald's 'On the therapeutic action of psychoanalysis' (Loewald, 1960) heralded such a change, at least in the USA. André Green's paper to the London Congress occupies a similar, pivotal position.

Anna Freud (1976) opened the discussion at the London Conference. She lent her enormous prestige as the daughter and heir to Sigmund Freud in support of Rangell's position. Her participation in the conference meant that the controversy would not be seen as taking place between Rangell and Green, but between Anna Freud and Green. She contrasted the foreboding atmosphere of that presentation of André Green's with the satisfaction and excitement that had characterised the attitude of the psychoanalytic pioneers. These pioneers felt that they were the first human beings privileged to understand the impact of the instinctual forces emanating from the unconscious mind. They were the first witnesses to a major revolution that was taking place in man's attempt to understand himself. In Anna Freud's opinion, psychoanalysis could fulfil its promise as long as it remained confined to patients with a potentially healthy ego suffering from neurotic symptoms. It is only within these confines that psychoanalysis can claim that its method of inquiry is identical with the cure. Neuroses imply normal development with average expectable mental structures, living within average expectable environments. When this optimal combination of forces is lacking, a very different developmental pathology takes place. Outside these limited conditions one cannot expect the success the psychoanalytic method promises. Instead of seeking to conquer new territories, Anna Freud counselled that we should recognise an 'optimum scope' for psychoanalytic therapy and use it only for what it can do best.

If we read Anna Freud's discussion at a distance of over twenty years, it is not so much that she disagreed with Green, but that she was unable to grasp what he was saying. In him she encountered a Freudian, but a Freudian who incorporated into his thinking ideas from Lacan, Bion and above all, from Winnicott. Green was keenly aware of the central position that symbolisation, or its absence, plays when one attempts to cure a borderline patient. This superstructure, going beyond Freud's formulation, seemed to Anna Freud a danger to Sigmund Freud's work, and unnecessary. Basically, for her, the development of psychoanalysis, at least at its core, ended with Sigmund Freud's formulations. In contrast to Anna Freud, Green took the invitation of the London Congress as an opportunity to create a new model to supplement Freud's model of neurosis as the negative of perversion. The new theoretical–clinical model was based on work with borderline patients. The model was created by Green, but he had absorbed into it what he learned from Lacan, Bion and Winnicott.

With André Green's (1975b) paper we were transplanted into a different world. Unlike traditional psychoanalysts, he approached the history of psychoanalysis dialectically. Psychoanalysis is going through a crisis. It is suffering from a deep malaise. There are contradictions between psychoanalysis and the social environment. There are contradictions at the very heart of psychoanalytic institutions. And finally, there are contradictions in the theory and practice of psychoanalysis itself. He emphasised that the optimistic self-satisfied attitude of the Hartmann era had given way to a greater complexity and a deepening anxiety.

André Green differentiated three lines of development that took place within psychoanalysis. The first centred its attention on inner conflict, the unconscious and points of fixation. It moved towards the study of the ego and its defence mechanisms. The second line of development moved towards object relations. The third gave priority to the function of the analytic setting, which in turn defines the analytic object. The first two groups are familiar. The third seems a creation of Green himself and came into being after psychoanalysts made the unwelcome discovery that some patients cannot use the analytic setting as a facilitating environment.

A variety of defence mechanisms, unsuspected by both Anna Freud (1936) and Otto Fenichel (1945), have been discovered and demand the attention of any psychoanalyst working with patients beyond the classical neuroses. Among these, Green enumerates somatic exclusion, expulsion via action, splitting and decathexis. 'Acting out' Green saw as the counterpart to psychosomatic 'acting in'. To these we should add splitting, emphasised by the Kleinians. Unlike American ego psychologists and Anna Freud (1972), Green takes the death instinct seriously. It finds expression in the decathexis of many vital interests: such patients aspire to attain a state of emptiness and non-being.

André Green defined decathexis in a way it had not traditionally been defined. In his formulation, decathexis takes place as a result of negative narcissism arising directly from the destructive instincts. Because of the power of the death instinct, ego cathexes are reduced to naught and negative narcissism becomes a force which 'decathects ego libido, without returning it to the object'. When this happens 'the ego becomes as disinterested in itself as in the object, leaving only a yearning to vanish: to be drawn towards death and Nothingness' (Green, 1986, p. 13).

Repression bars access from the unconscious to the conscious, but what has been repressed remains alive and seeks to return from repression. Thus, in spite of repression, the patient remains inwardly alive. By contrast, decathexis is deadlier, a mechanism before which the analyst is frequently helpless. It is no wonder that ego psychologists wished to close their eyes to its dangers. The paper on the dead mother (Green, 1983) could never have been written by Green had he not faced the deadly power of decathexis as a fundamental alternative to repression. Once the significance of this mechanism has been grasped, a new group of patients become accessible to psychoanalytic contact in the sense that they can feel that their therapist understands them and their plight, even if he or she cannot overcome the power of this deadly defence.

In another essay (1975a, pp. 292–3), we learn that the term decathexis was influenced by Winnicott's *Playing and Reality* (1971), where Winnicott described the work with severely disturbed patients. What takes place between analyst and analysand is a succession of libidinal aggressive cathexes and decathexes; the analysand destroys the analyst only to find that the analyst survives.

> The implicit model of neurosis in the past led us back to castration anxiety. The implicit model of these borderline states leads us back to the contradiction formed by the duality of separation anxiety/intrusion anxiety ... The patient then suffers from the combined effects of a persecutory intrusive object and of depression consequent on the loss of the object.
>
> (Green, 1975b, p. 7)

What is original and to many psychoanalysts disturbing in Green's approach is the idea that to understand the borderline patient, the analyst must include his own countertransference. What is difficult in our work with these patients is the polarity between delusion and death. Their psychotic core consists of a blank psychosis, a state without symptoms and psychic content. For these patients, the two parents are not differentiated from each other. Both are either bad and intrusive, or good and inaccessible.

The ego psychologists Fenichel (1974), Hartmann et al. (1949) and Anna Freud (1972) tried to protect psychoanalysis from the implications of the death instinct. It is of historical interest that Fenichel's paper was written in 1937 but was circulated only privately and could be published only posthumously in 1974. By contrast, Melanie Klein accepted the death instinct when she postulated that at the beginning of life there is the battle between the death instinct and Eros, which under favourable conditions promotes the development from the paranoid position to the depressive position.

I recall an analysand I saw many years ago whom I would now classify as belonging to this group. When I once asked him what was wrong with his previous analyst, he said, 'He was a good analyst for healthy patients, but not for me.' At that time I failed to understand the ominous meaning of that self-observation. In my own work I have found that analysands who have decathected their relationship to their inner bad objects nevertheless also fight the analyst in their own passive way by their continuous attack on linkage, a term we owe to Bion. They gracefully permit us to uncover one trauma after another because every trauma justifies their withdrawal from life; but they do not make use of this knowledge. They fail to integrate their biography in a new way that may give the life drive a chance to combat their tendency towards passivity and ultimately towards death.

I would now like to quote a few additional lines in which André Green presented his conclusions to the London Congress. To my knowledge, this had never been articulated within psychoanalysis before.

> The object which is always intrusively present, permanently occupying the personal psychic space, mobilizes a permanent counter-cathexis in order to combat this break-in, which exhausts the resources of the ego or forces it to get rid of its burden by expulsive projection. Never being absent it cannot be thought. Conversely, the inaccessible object can never be brought into the personal space, or at least never in a sufficiently durable way. This conflict leads to divine idealization which conceives of an inaccessible good object. The final result is paralysis of thought which is expressed in a negative hyper-chondriasis, particularly with regard to the head, i.e. a feeling of empty-headedness, of a whole mental activity, inability to concentrate, to remember, etc.
>
> (Green, 1975b, p. 8)

Juxtaposing the all-invasive bad object with the inaccessible good object which the analysand so ardently seeks and cannot find, not only gave psychoanalysts a new weapon in their struggle with severely disturbed men and women, it was also a contribution to the understanding of loving, and provided a new psychological understanding of the literature on mysticism and the history of religion. In normative religion, God is experienced as distant. Prayer may or may not reach him, and often requires an intermediary. By contrast, the mystic seeks ways to experience God physically and directly. Mysticism is a rebellion against the inaccessible good object.

At this point we also become acquainted with André Green's way of thinking dialectically. The object is bad, but it is good that it exists even though it does not exist as a good object. The abandonment of the bad object does not lead to the cathexis of a personal space, but to a tantalising aspiration towards nothingness which draws the patient down to a bottomless pit and eventually to a negative hallucination of the self.

Green concludes the paper with the observation that Freud's work has become the basis of our knowledge, but an analyst cannot practise psychoanalysis and keep it alive by merely applying existing knowledge. He must attempt to be creative to the limits of his ability. In my view, here Green has returned to one of the contradictions mentioned earlier in his paper, that operates at the heart of psychoanalytic institutions: Freud and the founders of the International implicitly accepted the idea that the majority of the practising psychoanalysts will apply to their patients what they learned at their Institute. We learn from Freud's letters to Abraham (1965) that both were convinced that the important discoveries had already been made, leaving to the next generation a kind of 'mopping-up' operation. Today we know that Freud did not fully understand the magnitude of his discoveries. Almost a hundred years after the great discoveries were made, André Green has shown in this paper that a vast territory still remains to be explored, and that the task Freud started proved to be infinitely more complex. One of the disturbing questions raised by Green goes to the very core of the psychoanalytic institutions. Must every analyst really be creative? Or is psychoanalysis like any other profession, capable of transmitting to its students a body of information that can give them the necessary security in their practice without burdening them with the need to be creative in the way they apply it?

The question of whether an analyst must be creative or merely well trained reflects a larger issue: whether analysands fall conveniently into a few diagnostic categories whose specific problems can be learned during training; or whether every analysand is unique and requires an individually tailored approach. If the latter is the case, then the practice of analysis demands a measure of creativity from every analyst. Psychoanalytic institutes, by their very structure, can only transmit acquired knowledge and cannot foster a creativity that is not part of the trained psychoanalyst's personality.

When we look back to the London debate twenty-eight years later, we can see that what was debated had historically already been decided. In the debate itself, Rangell and Anna Freud carried the day. But the era they represented had already passed. The USA was no longer the pace-setter for developments in psychoanalysis. Different schools challenged the wisdom of orthodox elders, and it was no longer possible to limit psychoanalytic efforts to neurotics only. In the interim, the treatment of neurotics has yielded no new information, and the insistence that psychoanalysis remain restricted to the treatment of neuroses contributed to the demise of the Hartmann era, even in the United States.

The concept of decathexis is also central to 'The dead mother' (Green, 1983). Green now singled out the greater emphasis on mourning as the most important characteristic that differentiates contemporary from earlier, classical analysis. The term dead mother is a metaphor, since the mother is physically alive. She had once been a source of vitality to her child, but because of a trauma suffered while the child was still young, she has withdrawn her interest and love from the child, 'brutally transforming a living object, which was a source of vitality for the child, into a distant figure, toneless, practically inanimate' (ibid., p.142). The period of mother's vitality must have been long enough to not have extinguished all hope for life in the child. In this respect, Green's dead mother patients differ from those studied by Spitz in his essays on hospitalism (Spitz, 1945, 1946).

In 'The dead mother', Green returned to some ideas expressed in the London Congress. The decathexis of the dead mother results in identification with her. Therefore, these patients experience no hatred for their mothers. These patients become attached to the analytic setting rather than to the analyst himself. The decathexis of the mother results in what Green calls 'psychological holes'. It is a technical error for the analyst to interpret the decathexis as a form of hatred. It can be considered a good omen when this blank depression becomes an experienced depression in the transference. Green speaks of a 'transference depression' in the way classical analysts spoke of transference neurosis.

In my own work with children of survivors I came across a variant on this theme, a mother who, over a stretch of time, is inanimate and then wakes up and is available for some time, only to succumb once again to her depression. Such babies or children have no way of understanding these fluctuations. They either identify with this mother and repeat this behaviour with their spouses and children, including the transference, or try by various techniques to keep the object from losing interest, at times maintaining both techniques alternately.

Discussion

Since the term decathexis is central to André Green's thinking, it may be useful to note that the term does not appear in Freud's *Standard Edition*, nor in the two major psychoanalytic dictionaries (Moore and Fine, (1990); Laplanche and Pontalis (1973)). The term cathexis was created by Strachey as a translation of the German *Besetzung*, a term Freud used to account for various degrees of intensity in which unconscious mental processes take place. The term then led to three additional terms, anticathexis and countercathexis and decathexis. When I encountered the term, it had a ring of familiarity for me, probably because my teacher Paul Federn had prepared me for André Green's idea in two papers, 'The ego as a subject and object in narcissism' (1928), and 'On the distinction between healthy and pathological narcissism' (1929). Federn attempted to use psychotics to arrive at a new model in a way similar to André Green's attempt to use borderline patients. In 1963 I pointed out that Federn's ego psychology was pushed aside by Hartmann's ego psychology.

In 1993, I suggested that the complexity of psychoanalysis itself demands that we differentiate between extenders, modifiers and heretics. As long as Freud was alive, there could be only loyal extenders and expelled heretics. After his death, inevitably, a third category had to emerge: that of modifiers. Once they appeared, psychoanalytic pluralism became inevitable. The historical moment for the emergence of modification was the crucial debate between Anna Freud and her followers, and Melanie Klein and her disciples. In this debate, Anna Freud was not powerful enough to expel the Kleinians from psychoanalysis. As a result, other modifiers, for example, Kohut and his followers, could also remain within organised psychoanalysis. That the same did not happen to Lacan and his followers is a subject that deserves special treatment. In my vocabulary, Lacan, Bion and Winnicott are examples of modifiers, and Green's effort at the London Congress was to unify three different modifiers as legitimate heirs to Freud's work.

In the same paper I also suggested that in view of the complexity of psychoanalysis, Freud's wish to be compared to Copernicus and Darwin as the third discoverer who disturbed the sleep of mankind, is not likely to come true. What is more likely is that Freud would be compared to Plato as one who gave rise to a complex history of ideas that would in time develop in many directions. The complexity of Freud's work is responsible for the fact that already there are many interpretations of its meaning. We recall that Melanie Klein proclaimed that she was a Freudian, but not an 'Anna Freudian'.

Within an historical perspective, it will be of interest to contrast the London debate with an earlier one, 'The widening scope of indications for psychoanalysis'. It was the subject matter of the Arden House conference in New York in 1954. The participants were Leo Stone, who presented his well-known paper on the subject. His presentation was followed by another classical paper by Edith Jacobson, entitled 'Transference problems in psychoanalytic treatment of severely depressive patients'. In that symposium, Anna Freud was the main discussant.

What strikes us forcibly when we read Stone's paper today is the change in the social atmosphere:

In a city like New York, scarcely any human problem admits of solution other than psychoanalysis: by the same token, there is an almost expectation of help from the method which does it grave
injustice. Hopeless or grave reality situations, lack of talent or ability
(usually regarded as an 'inhibition'), lack of adequate philosophy of
life, and almost any chronic physical illness may be brought to psychoanalysis for cure.

(Stone, 1954, p. 568)

Even when it was believed that psychoanalysis was a cure for every malady,
character disorders and borderline patients were frequently encountered in
psychoanalytic practice. Stone noted that the growing interest in ego
psychology resulted in the analyst paying greater attention to individual
nuances of character.

Stone devoted considerable energy to combating the idea that psychoanalysis can be harmful to any patient. A predisposition to psychosis does not
imply that a preformed psychosis exists in latent form in the adult, to appear
only because it is uncovered by the treatment. Stone concludes:

While the difficulties increase and the expectations of success dimin-
ish in a general way as the nosological periphery is approached, there
is no absolute barrier; and it is to be borne in mind that both extra-
nosological factors and the therapist's personal tendencies may profoundly influence the indication and prognosis.

(Stone, 1954, p. 593)

The success of treatment depends on the patient's capacity to tolerate
suffering, the capacity for self-observation and chronological age, occupation,
family milieu, and the rewards that can be reasonably expected to result from
intrapsychic change. Under favourable conditions a borderline patient may
profit more from psychoanalysis than some hysterics do. Stone goes on to
raise the question: 'How far can the classical analytical method be modified,
and still be regarded as psychoanalysis?' (ibid., p. 575)

Jacobson's paper is of interest in connection with Green's dead mother
syndrome. Both the similarities and the differences between the two papers
are instructive. Jacobson pointed out that depressives try to recover their lost
ability to love through the magic love they hope to receive from their love-
objects. They tend to establish either an immediate intense rapport, or none.
This makes it risky to refer them to another therapist. Their transference is
characterised by exaggerated idealisation and an obstinate denial of visible
shortcomings of their analyst. They often feel better without any apparent
intrapsychic reasons. The mere hope that analysis will cure them is sufficient
to bring about improvement in their feelings. They tend to make heavy
demands on their analysts.

Much more depends on the emotional quality in the analyst's responses than on the quantity of sessions. Many depressives tolerate four or even three sessions weekly much better than six or seven ... Daily sessions may be experienced as seductive promises too great to be fulfilled, or then again as intolerable oral sadistic obligations which promote the masochistic submission.

(Jacobson, 1954, p. 603)

Jacobson goes on to say that these patients need the analyst, mainly as a tolerant listener to their repetitive complaints. It is helpful to these patients when during the period of positive transference the analyst draws their attention to the illusory nature of the transference. When the transference becomes negative, one must avoid interpretations. During this phase, any interpretation by the analyst is experienced as a defensive behaviour, and as his unavailability to the patient's need. If we read Jacobson's paper with Green's Dead Mother in mind, we see that her patients have not reached the state of decathexis that Green's patients have experienced. Or, if they did, Jacobson was not cognisant of that aspect of their experience.

In Anna Freud's discussion of these two papers, she regretted that so much interest is withdrawn from the treatment of traditional neurosis. She stated:

If all the skill, knowledge, and pioneering effort which was spent in widening the scope of application of psychoanalysis had been employed instead on intensifying and improving our technique in the original field, I cannot help but feel that by now, we would find the treatment of common neuroses child's play, instead of struggling with their technical problems, as we have continued to do.

(A. Freud, 1954, p. 610)

If we read this statement today, we discern something that was never fully faced: namely, that Anna Freud – and she must be looked upon as typical of many analysts of the time – was looking forward to an era in which psychoanalysis would become what she called 'child's play', a work that can be done by any reasonably well-trained practitioner.

If we compare the 1954 symposium with that of 1975, we note that Stone and Jacobson speak to a confident, optimistic psychoanalytic audience. In fact, the therapeutic successes of psychoanalysis at that time were modest. But this fact had little effect on the optimism and the high expectations regarding what psychoanalysis can deliver. It seems that, like Jacobson's depressive patients, psychoanalysts lived on hope. For its part, the London symposium took place in an atmosphere of uncertainty and doubt. The enthusiasm of the pioneers had given way to the professionalisation of psychoanalysis. Psychoanalysis had become a difficult profession to follow, requiring (at least, in the USA) years of training beyond the MD, and psychiatric training as well. All too many analysts had made the painful discovery that their own training analyses had left much to be desired. At the same time, the worlds of literature and entertainment, once so enthusiastic about psychoanalysis, had become indifferent or even hostile. Furthermore, psychoanalysis itself was no longer a unified movement. Modifiers had created different schools, and these were at war with each other. The centre, so eloquently defended by Rangell and Anna Freud, could not turn back the tide of change that André Green had represented.

The command of the Delphic oracle, for man to know himself, turned out to be infinitely harder to execute than the psychoanalytic pioneers envisioned; but the road to that goal proved more interesting than these pioneers foresaw. And one of the important markers on that road was André Green's discovery of decathexis as an alternative to repression.

References

Abraham, H. and Freud, E. (eds) (1965) *A Psycho-Analytic Dialogue: The Letters of Sigmund Freud and Karl Abraham, 1907–1926*. New York: Basic Books.

Bergmann, M. S. (1963) The place of Paul Federn's ego psychology in psychoanalytic metapsychology. *Journal of the American Psychoanalytic Association* 11: 97–116.

—— (1993) Psychoanalytic education and the social reality of psychoanalysis. *Psychoanalytic Review* 80/2: 199–210.

—— (1999) *An Evaluation of the Hartmann Era*. New York: The Other Press.

Bergmann, M. S. and Hartman, F. (1976) *The Evolution of Psychoanalytic Technique*. New York: Columbia University Press.

Federn, P. (1928) The ego as subject and object in narcissism. In W. Weiss (ed.) *Ego Psychology and the Psychoses*. New York: Basic Books (1952).

—— (1929) On the distinction between healthy and pathological narcissism. In W. Weiss (ed.) *Ego Psychology and the Psychoses*. New York: Basic Books (1952).

Fenichel, O. (1945) *The Psychoanalytic Theory of Neurosis*. New York: W. W. Norton.

—— (1974) A review of Freud's 'Analysis Terminable and Interminable'. *The International Review of Psycho-Analysis* 1: 109–16.

Freud, A. (1936) *The Ego and the Mechanisms of Defense*. New York: International Universities Press.

—— (1954) The widening scope of indications for psychoanalysis: discussions. *Journal of the American Psychoanalytic Association* 2: 607–20.

—— (1972) Comments on aggression. *International Journal of Psycho-Analysis* 53: 163–71.

—— (1976) Changes in psychoanalytic practice and experience. *International Journal of Psycho-Analysis* 57: 257–60.

Green, A. (1975a) Potential space in psychoanalysis: the object in setting. In *On Private Madness*. Madison, CT: International Universities Press, 1986.

—— (1975b) The analyst, symbolization and the absence in the analytic setting (on changes in analytic practice and analytic experience). *International Journal of Psycho-Analysis* 56: 1–22. Also in *On Private Madness*. Madison, CT: International Universities Press.

—— (1983) The dead mother. In *On Private Madness*. Madison, CT: International Universities Press, 1986.

—— (1986) Introduction. In *On Private Madness*. Madison, CT: International Universities Press.

Hartmann, H. (1939) *Ego Psychology and the Problem of Adaptation*. New York: International Universities Press, (1958).

Hartmann, H., Kris, E. and Loewenstein, R. (1949) Notes on the theory of aggression. *Psychological Issues* (1964) 4(2): 56–85.

Jacobson, E. (1954) Transference problems in the psychoanalytic treatment of severely depressive patients. *Journal of the American Psychoanalytic Association* 2: 595–606.

King, P. and R. Steiner (eds) (1991) *The Freud–Klein Controversies, 1941–1945*. London: Tavistock/Routledge.

Laplanche, J. and Pontalis, J. (1973) *The Language of Psychoanalysis*. (Translated by D. Nicholson-Smith.) New York: W. W. Norton.

Loewald, Hans W. (1960) On the therapeutic action of psycho-analysis. *International Journal of Psycho-Analysis* 41: 16–33.

Marienbad Symposium on the theory of the therapeutic results of psycho-analysis. (1937) Papers by E. Glover, O. Fenichel, J. Strachey, E. Bergler, N. Nunberg and E. Bibring. *International Journal of Psycho-Analysis* 38: 125–88.

Moore, B. and Fine, B. (1990) *Psychoanalytic Terms and Concepts*. New Haven: Yale University Press.

Rangell, L. (1975) Psychoanalysis and the process of change: an essay on the past, present and future. *International Journal of Psycho-Analysis* 56: 87–98.

Shengold, L. and McLaughlin, J. T. (reporters) (1976) Plenary session on 'Changes in psychoanalytic practice and experience: theoretical, technical and social implications'. *International Journal of Psycho-Analysis* 57: 261–74.

Spitz, R. A. (1945) Hospitalism. *Psychoanalytic Study of the Child* 1: 53–74.

—— (1946) Hospitalism: a follow-up report. *Psychoanalytic Study of the Child* 2: 113–17.

Stone, L. (1954) The widening scope of indications for psychoanalysis. *Journal of the American Psychoanalytic Association* 2: 567–620.

Winnicott, D. W. (1971) *Playing and Reality*. London: Tavistock Publications.

11

THE INTUITION OF THE NEGATIVE IN *PLAYING AND REALITY*

André Green

In 1993, I introduced a new concept, *Le Travail du négatif* (The work of the negative) which became the title of a book published at the time (Green, 1993a). In the introductory chapter of this book, I declared that one of the sources that guided me in my elaboration was Winnicott, to whom I was indebted – specifically to his *Playing and Reality*.[1] Nevertheless, if one turns to two recent dictionaries on Winnicott's work, written by Alexander Newman (1995) and Jan Abram (1996), there is no mention in them of the negative.

Let us go back to *Playing and Reality*. In the first sentence of the Introduction, Winnicott writes: 'This book is the development of my paper "Transitional objects and transitional phenomena" (1951)'.[2] If we read that article carefully we shall be able to find the thread, whether apparent or invisible, which runs through the whole book. In fact, this paper has a particular history. It is dated 1951, in its initial version. This text will later be the first chapter of *Playing and Reality* in 1971, in a modified form bearing the same title. The 1951 paper appears in 1971 as the first section of the chapter under another title: 'Original hypothesis',[3] with two new sections entitled: 'II. An application of the theory', and 'III. Clinical material: aspects of fantasising', in which the negative is introduced. Section II had already been published in 1960 and 1965, separately. This section starts with a few lines of introduction followed by a sub-section: 'Psychopathology manifested in the area of transitional phenomena'. The beginning of this sub-section substantially modifies the last lines of the 1951–53 paper in which Winnicott wrote initially about the application of his ideas in psychopathology, that is, 'addiction, fetishism and pseudologia fantastica and thieving'. In *Playing and Reality*, these applications are suppressed and instead Winnicott focuses on separation and loss. He brings the idea of a limited tolerance to separation in terms of the duration of the separation from the mother object. He continues with a clinical example, entitled 'String'.[4] Section II of *Playing and Reality* ends with an 'added note 1969', which is included here in this new context, published posthumously in the book.

Much of what I will have to say is borrowed from the clinical material (section III), which is entirely new, in this last version of the paper. But there is a long preparatory phase to the new ideas of the book that is already present in the 1951 paper, before the explicit idea of the negative develops and is integrated in this seminal paper. The clinical material is supposed to show 'how the sense of loss itself can become a way of integrating one's self-experience' (1971, p. 20). Here, the explicit references to the negative have to do with a pathological structure, but in my view there are other aspects of the notion in the paper, which are linked with Winnicott's ideas on normal development and can be found in the beginning of the chapter and in the 1951 version of the paper.

For example, defining the transitional object as 'not-me' possession proposes an angle to the concept of object different from its usual positive connotations either as a need satisfying object, an object of desire or as a phantasised object. The object is here defined as a negative of me, which has many implications with regard to omnipotence. To distinguish between the first object and the first 'not-me' possession, as Winnicott does, extends our thinking, especially if this is located in an intermediate area between two parts of two bodies, mouth and breast, which will create some third object in between them, not only in the actual space that separates them, but in the potential space of their reunion after their separation. This, also, because it implies the idea of something that is not present, is another meaning of the negative. This notion of a 'third' object has its application in the analytic situation. I have proposed that we understand the exchanges between patient and analyst or, in other terms, between transference and countertransference processes, as creating an 'analytic third', a specific outcome of analysis (Green, 1975, pp. 1–22; reprinted in 1986). This idea has been developed since by Ogden (1994a, b) and Gabbard (1997).

The creation of the transitional object is important: 'not so much the object used as the use of the object' (1971, p. xii). Winnicott here alludes to the paradox involved in that use, a paradox (as he said) that has to be accepted, tolerated and respected without forced attempts to solve it. That paradox – no attention has been paid to this – includes a tolerance of the negative, as is mentioned in his section on symbolism. Winnicott writes: 'It's not being the breast (or the mother), although real, is as important as the fact that it stands for the breast' (1971, p. 6). Let us notice, in this same section, an expression of great significance: opposing fantasy and fact, internal and external objects, primary creativity and perception, he states that the term transitional object refers to symbolism *in time*. It describes the infant's journey from the purely subjective to objectivity; and it seems to me that the transitional object (piece of blanket, teddy bear, etc.) is what we see of this *journey of progress towards experiencing* (p. 14, my italics).

Instead of being tempted to focus on the opposite terms, which is what any fast reader of Winnicott will be tempted to do, or even on the space between them, I shall draw our attention to the idea of the journey. I will come back to it later. The journey expresses the dynamic quality of the experience, implying a move in the space linked with time. I shall dare to suggest that Winnicott develops here an alternative to Freud's theory of the drive that includes a similar dynamic dimension and a similar change in the space from the source to the object. Let us remember, the transitional space is not just 'in between'; it is a space where the future subject is *in transit*, taking possession of a created object in the vicinity of a real external one, before he has reached it.

From this conception of normal development, Winnicott's work focuses progressively on another conception of the negative. Until then the negative was a quality inherent in psychic functioning, for instance, not–me possession, the paradox of not being and being the breast as well and at the same time being a substitute for it, not being an internal object or an external one but a 'possession', etc. From now on, Winnicott is going to describe some pathological issues which need a 'complex statement' (1971, p. 9).[5] 'The infant can employ a transitional object when the internal object is alive and real and good enough (not too persecutory). But this internal object depends for its qualities on the existence and aliveness and behaviour of the external object. *Failure of the latter in some essential function indirectly leads to deadness or to a persecutory quality of the internal object*' (p. 9).[6] After a persistence of inadequacy of the external object, the internal object fails to have meaning to the infant, and then, and only then does the transitional object become meaningless too (pp. 9–10).

In the 1951 paper, Winnicott gives the example of two brothers, the elder, X, having failed to form a transitional object. He has an early and persistent attachment to the mother herself. Though he could adopt a rabbit (a toy), the object never had the quality of a transitional object. So it is not only the presence or the absence of an object that looks like a transitional one which is meaningful, but the presence or absence of the signs that indicate its quality as such. Winnicott points out that he never married. His younger brother Y, sucked his thumb, weaned without difficulty, adopted the blanket, used the wool to tickle his nose, invented words to designate his blanket and is now a father. Both are 'normal' but the differences are striking. These remarks pave the way to the added sections of the paper in the *Playing and Reality* version devoted to psychopathology. Winnicott then seems to understand – in contrast to what he wrote in his 1951 paper where the notion is scarcely mentioned – the prime importance of absence in the psychopathology of the transitional area. He writes:

If the mother is away over a period of time which is beyond a certain limit measured in minutes, hours, or days, then the memory of the internal representation fades. As this takes effect, the transitional phenomena become gradually meaningless and the infant is unable to experience them. '*We may watch the object becoming decathected.*'

(p. 15, my italics)

This fading of the internal representations is what I relate to the inner representation of the negative, 'a representation of the absence of representation', as I say, which expresses itself in terms of negative hallucination, or in the field of affects, in terms of a void, emptiness or, to a lesser degree, futility, meaninglessness.

These observations precede the beautiful, moving and finally tragic example of the string, which I will not comment on again here. The omnipresence of the string in the child's play – a squiggle game played with Winnicott – led him to a conclusion about his little patient that he communicated to the mother: 'I explained to the mother that this boy was dealing with a fear of separation, attempting to deny separation by his use of a string, as one would deny separation from a friend by using the telephone' (ibid., p. 17). This was an explanation that the mother found silly but that, on second thought, she could use. The string was a positive materialisation of an absent, negative bond.

In the footnote added in 1969, Winnicott sadly confesses, a decade after the case was first reported, that the child could not be cured of his illness. The denial of his fear of separation was not only linked with his mother's absence while she was hospitalised but also and even more with the absence of contact with her when she was physically present.[7] 'She [the mother] made the very significant comment that she felt the most important separation to have been his loss of her when she was seriously depressed; it was not just her going away, she said, but her lack of contact with him because of her complete preoccupation with other matters' (ibid., p. 17). In consequence, the child would never accept physical separations from the mother later on. The whole case should be reported in detail.

We are now ready to come to the more explicit idea of the negative, referring to the last section of the chapter. Until now we have had to deduce the notion from the text – from now on, as we will see, the notion will be openly expressed.

Winnicott uses the material from *one* session of an adult patient, a woman. The patient starts by reporting a dream in which *the present analyst is seen as an avaricious dominating woman*, which leads her to regret a former analyst seen as a male figure for her. She fantasises intensely – about catastrophic anxieties related to journeys – on the impossibility of letting other people know what misfortunes beset her; on being heard crying or screaming, the object being always out of reach. Winnicott states: 'Much of the material in this analysis has to do with coming to the negative side of relationships' (ibid., p. 21). This included the patient's own experience as a child, and experiences with her children, whom she had to leave for a holiday. On her return she was told that the child had cried for four hours. Winnicott interprets the situation as traumatic, as no explanation can be given to a 2-year-old child, or to a cat for the absence of the mother. This leads to an experience where the mother is 'dead' from the point of view of the baby. After an amount of time, the mother is definitely dead, whether absent or present. This means no contact can be re-established when she is back. 'This is what dead means,' says Winnicott. Winnicott's work is here very close to mine in my description of the dead mother (1983). It is important to link two extremes, which are very different: 'the death of the mother when she is present and her death when she is able to reappear and therefore to come alive again' (1971, p. 22). The separation is irreversible and the tendency to re-experience it as strong as the manifestation of a drive in repetition compulsion.

During World War II, the patient, age 11, was evacuated (very far away from her home). She completely forgot her childhood. But, on the other hand, she was strongly opposed to calling the people who took care of her 'uncle' or 'auntie', as the other children did in their new families. 'She managed *never to call them anything*,' says Winnicott, 'and this was the *negative of remembering* her mother and father' (ibid., p. 22) [my italics].

These many examples of the negative show how Winnicott was close to a notion that he never had a chance to promote to a theoretical status. Nor did his readers. This all refers to a lack: absence of memory, absence in the mind, absence of contact, absence of feeling alive – all these absences can be condensed in the idea of a gap. But that gap, instead of referring to a simple void or to something which is missing, becomes the substratum for what is real. Winnicott says that the only real thing is the gap: 'that is to say the death, the absence or the amnesia' (ibid., p. 22). When the patient experiences an important amnesia during the session, Winnicott writes that:

> the important communication for me to get was that there could be a blotting out, and that this blank could be the only fact and the only thing that was real. The amnesia is real, whereas what is only forgotten has lost its reality.
>
> (ibid., p. 22)

One can easily make the difference here between what has been blotted out, or, in my own terms, has undergone a negative hallucination, and what is only forgotten, or, in Freud's terms, repressed.

At one point in the session, the patient remembers that there is a rug in the consulting room that she once used to cover herself with in a period of regression. But now she won't use it any more. 'The reason is that the rug that is not there (because she does not go for it) is more real than the rug the analyst might bring, as he certainly had the idea to do' (ibid., p. 22). I would add that not using the rug is an absolute necessity. It is a fact to which she will come back at the end of the session, when leaving Winnicott, telling him that the rug could be comfortable, but reality is more important than comfort. She shows also that using the rug would be a sign of forgiveness or that reparation has occurred. If so, the reality of the revenge would fade. But this is mine, not Winnicott's.

In the end, the patient's attitude culminates in the idea that the former analyst (of whom she complained so much) will always be more important to her than the present one (himself). The patient is able to recognise that Winnicott does her more good, but has to confess that she likes the former better. The patient produces here one of those sentences (which not unlike those of Freud) are a kind of seal to characterise a situation. 'The negative of him is more real than the positive of you' (ibid., p. 23). In her elaboration, the patient would say: 'I suppose I want something that never goes away' (ibid., p. 23). This is obvious, but what is missing here is that the bad object is the one that never goes away. *And the bad thing, whether present or absent, is negative anyway in two ways: as bad and as non-existent.* The judgement of attribution and the judgement of existence coincide. The bad thing has to be there, and if it is not, it is this absence equated with void and emptiness that becomes real, more real than the existing objects that are around. 'The real thing is the thing that is not here' (ibid., p. 24).

The patient was highly gifted intellectually. From the very beginning, Winnicott tells her that the use of her intellect reflects a fear of mental defect. In fact, the symbols she uses could be real for a time, but in the end they fade away. There were reasons to think that she had been anxious because of the appearance of a schizophrenic condition in her environment.

One could see how this concern was linked with uncontrolled aggression and threat of disintegration. Instead, the patient had organised devices to master the destruction. The patient told Winnicott that she used to pull the legs off a paper spider every day her mother was away – a spider that could be used like a daisy, to test love. On the other hand, denial of separation could be seen in her relatives. The mother of the patient, wanting her child to feel guilty for always complaining and bothering her, told her that when she was 21/2 years old: 'we "heard" you cry all the time we were away' (ibid., p. 24) – that is, four miles away. She could not admit her mother was lying to her; maybe she thought she was omnipresent. It could give her the feeling that she was not separated from her, if she still heard her.

Symbolisation was obviously present but needed to be understood specifically. There was much evidence of its manifestations. But, as Winnicott says, the patient gradually had '*to doubt the reality of the thing that they* [the transitional objects] *were symbolising*' (ibid., p. 24).

All her life, the patient was haunted by the fear of losing animals, her own children, all her possessions. This was formulated in the sentence: 'All I have got is what I have not got' (ibid.). Winnicott comments: 'The negative is the only positive' (ibid.). When asked by the patient what he would do about it, Winnicott first remained mute and then said: 'I am silent because I don't know what to say' (ibid.), an answer that pleased the patient, probably because the analyst confessed his impotence. It also recognised her ability to protect her mind from his intrusiveness, which led to a triumph of annihilating him.

All this material comes from one session. At the end of it, leaving the analyst and having to go on a railway journey to her holiday house, she expressed the idea that Winnicott could come with her, halfway. After a while the separation would no longer matter. She mocked Winnicott's maternal identification and imagined him on the train overwhelmed by a lot of babies and children climbing over him, vomiting on him, which was what he deserved. It is evident that she used him to project on him all the bad objects that she had contained during the session, and that she could imagine spitting out after the session, during the journey to her holiday house. She finally said that when she was evacuated during the war she went to that other country, wanting to see if her parents were there. She seemed to have believed she would find them there. Only after a year or two did she realise that they were not there and 'that was reality' (ibid., p. 5).

While I was preparing this paper, I remembered that I had in my notes the clinical material of a session with a patient that I presented in a seminar on the *travail du négatif*, in 1987, long before I wrote my book. I went back to it. Before reporting the session, I need to give a few words of explanation about my meeting with the patient. During the year I taught at University College, London, a lady asked to see me. She had attended my inaugural lecture and remembered that she had been advised to see me by one of her friends. The friend told her she had to see me because I was a kind of French Winnicott, a compliment I was far from deserving. This patient told me she had been in treatment with Winnicott for some years. She had abandoned the treatment with him, and some time later Winnicott died. She was very distressed not to be able to continue with anyone else after several failed attempts.

She had had her first analysis when she was young, making a lot of sacrifices and considerable efforts; but the analysis ended very badly, in a negative therapeutic reaction. The treatment was stopped by the analyst, who had had enough of her. Before finding Winnicott, she had been to a lot of analysts and therapists of all kinds, whom she abandoned sooner or later. And finally, she found Winnicott. She obviously had an extraordinary impression of their meetings; she used to tell me: 'No one is like Winnicott', which I was very ready to believe.

After our meeting, she seemed to be willing to ask me for some help, though we both knew it was impossible to have a proper analysis with me, as we lived in different towns. Even at the time I was teaching in London, I travelled back and forth each week from Paris to London. So, after having interviewed her a few times, I proposed that I would see her for a week or so, three or four times a year. I knew that, especially with this kind of patient, it was very inappropriate and that she would suffer a lot from our separation. But I had the feeling the contact that we had during these first interviews was of a sufficient quality (today I would say that I had been 'seduced') and could possibly be used during our encounters to help her understand what was going on with herself. In any case, it seemed impossible for me to refuse to help her, which she could only experience as a rejection. She accepted what I proposed, and what I had predicted happened. Being in an intense state of suffering in her chronic depressive illness, and also because I could not see her at the time, I suggested that she should see someone in London in the meanwhile. She tried to make an arrangement with the colleague I highly recommended but, for all sorts of reasons, things could not be worked out. This was both because of her very negative feelings towards him and also because he wouldn't accept the situation that placed him in the position of an intermittent substitute therapist, as she didn't mean to stop the relationship with me.

I realised afterwards that I had made a mistake, proposing a solution that neither of them was prepared to accept. It took me some time to realise that my patient was the one Winnicott wrote about in the last section of 'The transitional object and the transitional phenomena' paper published in *Playing and Reality*. Re-reading that section, I felt in total agreement with everything Winnicott said. I had the great luck of having a living experience of what was described in the paper – a chance that I felt was unique. There was no disagreement with anything I had read, only regrets that Winnicott did not state some facts that seemed very important to me, and to which I will come back later. I will present material from one session I had with this patient ten years ago, at least fifteen years after the one reported in Winnicott's book.

The patient would be very concerned to be totally isolated with me. She would start at any noise, couldn't bear to hear the bell ring or the telephone. She seemed in a state of terror, but I also felt terrorised by her reactions. She seemed to be confused, looking all around her, as if everything was strange. She wouldn't lie on the couch or sit on the chair in front of me; she sat on the couch and would start the session by saying: 'Where am I? What time is it? What am I doing here?' Then, after a silence, she would begin to speak.

'Let me tell you a dream. *My first analyst comes to visit me. After a while I think he's going to leave, but I realise that he won't. So, I have to cope with that situation and then I bend over him to kiss him*'. [This was the analyst whose negative was more real than the positive of Winnicott. I had some idea that at the beginning of the session I might represent him. But I was not so sure he was truly a male figure for her.] She continued, saying that after that dream I called to tell her that she could come to see me. [She had phoned earlier to see if this was possible and I had had to check before giving her a positive response.] 'One thing that makes me happy is that I gave up all my therapies [drugs] and I feel much better'.

A: You do not need any therapy to come to see me.
P: Yes. But what am I doing?
A: Continuing something, maybe.

P: Oh yes, I suppose this must be true. I think that many of my problems have to do with a situation about which something I say is here and with something else which is there, and there is between these two things a space in which something happens like travelling, going there and coming back. What can I do to go from here to there? Who is here and who is there? And above all, how do I come back?

You will easily recall how these words remind us of what Winnicott said in terms of facts and events. But here the patient is speaking of a mental state coinciding with her visiting me. It is also about the link between Winnicott and me. We can think that coming to Paris to see me can also be associated by her to the period where she was evacuated abroad. But even more, I pinpoint the metaphor of the journey as characterising what goes on in the intermediate area between subjective creativity and objective reality. An important concern is about being able to come back. In other terms, not to be lost in some desert, or in the middle of the ocean. The Greeks had a dread: of losing the way back. In fact, here she seems to be lost in the middle, not reaching anywhere. She told me about the risk of those children dying during the journey (because of the German attacks). After having stayed there for three years, she had changed so much, physically and morally, that her mother had not recognised her when she came back home, as if her mother too had lost her.

She continued:

I had an interesting experience: I have met two friends who were with me during the evacuation. They loved my mother and one has even said: 'How I wish she could be my mother!' She always had a photograph of my mother with her. For me she was such an awful, horrible mother, I could not understand. Well, I have been told that my mother did not behave with her own children as she did with the children of others. She must have been so different with them than with me.

I told her that this could also have something to do with the 'here' and 'there': 'Maybe it was as if you were not sure that you were the same person in the two places, "here" and "there". Just as it is difficult for you to bring together the two mothers, the mother who is with the others and your own mother.'

P: Yes. I have no memory before my leaving. But I have the impression that when I was there, in the country of the evacuation, it was as if my heart was plucked out and put aside and that life had continued. When I came back at 15, I had curled hair, my lips were painted, and I wore high heels. She did not recognise me.

A: Many things can change between 12 and 15.

P: Oh yes, of course; I had my periods. But that hadn't changed anything for me. I'm going to tell you something which I'm sure you don't know. Elizabeth Taylor has just written a book and appeared on television. She lost two stones and she has given up everything: drinking, treatment and the rest [This reminded me of her giving up drugs]. Can you imagine: I had a dream. During the war, every week we had an afternoon tea to which we invited soldiers and danced with them. And she, Elizabeth Taylor, in the dream, danced with my mother. Strange, isn't it. It is as if I couldn't leave my parents. When I think of them I have the feeling they beseech me: 'Please, allow us to leave, let us go'. But it is as if I couldn't.

A: Yes, that's the problem with losing two stones. [What I was alluding to were the two graves of her parents, and communicating to her that it was her parents' body in her own body.]

P: I never understand what you say. [She used to say that either about what she called my 'Freudian interpretations' or about the metaphorical style of them.] In fact, when I think of my mother in me, it is as if she is petrified. And the more time goes by, the more I am confronted with the necessity of accepting my parents' death, and the more there is something in me which cannot admit they exist no more. It is as if I held them as prisoners in a sort of purgatory or in limbo. [Her parents have been dead a long time.]

A   I think I remember that limbo is the place where dead babies remain. [She and her mother have lost babies.]

P: Oh yes. Non-baptised children.

She goes on, talking of her first pregnancy, which ended in a miscarriage. The fact that she had been pregnant was taken very badly by her family.

In the session, we could witness once again the deep link between her mother and herself, as her mother too had a stillborn baby, before the patient's own birth. She says, about her own dead child, that never will she be able to consider him as no longer existing. Again, mourning is impossible; there is a mutual persecution between her and the dead.

P: I have the feeling that my problem is all a question of space and time. But I feel a little bit better because I don't hang on to my therapists any more, insisting on them making me feel good. I understand that I must not ask them that any more. But going and coming back still raises problems. I cannot travel freely, because I always have to make sure when I travel that I can go to the loo. If I have to make a journey in a bus that has no loo, then I give up. All my thinking tries to connect: 'I go there, I take a connection here, I arrive there, I do this, I do that. I can only leave this way.'

She was looking for a place in the transitional area where she could deposit parts of her body, as if the bond between her and her mother was always there. (Winnicott made the remark that faeces could also be understood as transitional objects.)

The comparison between the two sessions is striking. One will be struck by the significant place of sexuality in the exchange with me, and its total absence with Winnicott. This is not only due to the difference in the transference. In fact, one can ask oneself if there was not an important censorship on sexuality in Winnicott's paper. In the 1951 version of the 'Transitional object' paper, there is a substantial discussion of Wulff's paper: 'Fetishism and object choice in early childhood' (1946), in which Winnicott considers the relationship of fetishism and the transitional object. This useful discussion disappears from the version published in *Playing and Reality*. The patient had been married to a sexually disturbed man from whom she was now divorced (Winnicott does not say anything about that; is it only for reasons of confidentiality?). She interrupted her analysis in order to have a love affair. This could not be excluded from the transference relationship. Moreover, during adolescence she had a very intense emotional relationship with her father who recognised her femininity, causing jealous reactions in her mother. But she resented her father because he did not fully appreciate her intellectual abilities. It does not seem right to me to consider these aspects of the material as a simple defence or even as irrelevant or of no importance. When she came to me, she commented that people in the hotel where she was staying had intimated that she came to Paris to see a lover. But, in fact, in the Elizabeth Taylor dream she represents a homosexual relationship with her mother. I suppose Elizabeth Taylor represented the 15-year-old girl coming back, expecting to seduce her mother. In fact, she was rebuked by her. If there was no dream, I would be tempted to consider this as superficial material. But it is clearly shown that the sexual transference to her first analyst is followed by the homosexual fantasy of dancing with her mother.

There is also a journey in the girl's sexual development in what Freud calls the change of object from mother to father. Anyhow, the elements of Winnicott's session are still there. The reference to the journey, to the amnesia, to the feeling of having lost her parents, mainly her mother, and above all, the idea of the journey associated to her being two different persons, at the start and in the end, the losing of the sense of continuity, the unacceptance of death, as if the bodies of her parents, and especially of her mother, were petrified in the cage of her own body (dead incorporations), all this still refers to the work of the negative and the considerable pain of investing positively the relationship with others. This patient would wake up in the morning and spend a long time moaning: 'I can't, I can't, I can't' for hours before she could get out of bed. The model of the journey seems to be like a dynamic representation of herself; a kind of ultimate attempt to fight the impression of dying in the gap or the void, recalling many things about which she complained at the beginning of our encounters.

During one of our separations, her cat escaped from the house, crossed the street, was hit by a car, and died. She felt an intense pain and wrote to me about what had happened. There were suggestions that the crushed cat lying on the ground could look like an abortion or even faeces. I could perfectly understand what that meant for her. In her letters, when she described the corpse of the poor cat, I could not avoid feeling that there was a kind of unconscious satisfaction, of which I think she was totally unaware. If I had interpreted this, I believe our relationship would have ended. Obviously the dead cat was a mother-baby animal. The accident happened while she was away. So it was her fault, as it was her mother's about what might have happened to her. Is one the same after having travelled so far?

In the work I have done with her, I have tried to take up again everything about her relationship with her mother that was worked through with Winnicott. But I progressively introduced the relationship with the father with all its related gratifications of eroticism and cultural exchange, from which her mother was excluded. Her intellectual activity was obviously driven by an identification with the father. We went as far as we could under the circumstances. She even managed to come for nearly a month, in order to have intensive treatment, though I warned her that I didn't feel I was omnipotent enough to cure her with that kind of magic therapy. But I am struck by the comparison of what she said to Winnicott at the end of the session he reports and what she had said to me, travelling on the metro and being confronted with the vomiting of some passengers and going back to London. In fact, as Winnicott told her once, it was as if she had never eaten anything. That infuriated her; she stopped the session and left.

At any event, she came for some years, less and less frequently, until she stopped seeing me because she did not feel the need to come any more. She always sends me postcards at Christmas, ironically, 'as all polite English people do'. She was still travelling a lot, but felt better, though not entirely free of symptoms.

Paradoxically, there is more in Winnicott's clinical material about my ideas on the negative than in my own session. Or, to put it differently, it is more explicitly shown in Winnicott's presentation. There are many reasons for that. Maybe the patient was more disturbed when she had that session with Winnicott than when she had hers with me. Maybe, also, because Winnicott wrote that chapter having in mind his ideas on the negative, which unfortunately he did not have the time to develop. As for myself, I only wrote the book *Le travail du négatif* some five years later and did not use the session for that purpose. But in both sessions, Winnicott's and mine, I have tried to link the normal aspects of the negative with the pathological ones. In Winnicott, the normal aspects are shown in the transitional objects. The first 'not me' possession, the paradox of being and not being the breast, etc. In my own case, I tried to reinterpret basic concepts of psychoanalysis to show how the negative is implicit in them.

For instance, the unconscious implies a reference to the negative, not only because it is not conscious, but also because, in Freud's descriptions, when he thinks of the relationship between two conscious representations in a free association context, he has to postulate the existence of an unconscious thought or representation between them. Here the negative is associated with the idea of the latent operating behind the scenes, invisible though active. One can even refer to a meaning that would make us think of a photograph, the negative being the element through which the positive can appear. Moreover, apart from this explicit example, certain other concepts refer to a similar structure. I think here of identification, seen, in some instances, as the opposite of an object relationship. Or, to put it more clearly, that there could be an opposition between, on the one hand, all the relationships based on desire, or implying a bodily contact (which I think would deserve to be called positive), and on the other, the processes operating on distant relationships with no contact except the one established in the mind, as in identification. In this last instance, the processes could be categorised as belonging to the negative. These are just a few examples of how the negative can be present in very ordinary concepts.

What we have to keep in mind is that in Freud's theory of the drives there is always an implication of something in excess in the psychic apparatus which has to be reduced or repressed or, I would say, 'negativated'. This applies to Freud's statement according to which neurosis is the negative of perversion. Winnicott's references are different because he is concerned mainly with separation, a phenomenon that occurs in normal as well as in pathological development. He is oriented mainly towards the object, while I consider the situation from the point of view of the presence of the drives. Anyhow, the reference to absence (common to Lacan and Winnicott) is directly related to the negative as that which is not present; not positively perceived through the senses.

I will propose another model that will account for the normal, 'positive' aspects of the negative. When we think of the early mother–child relationship, in Winnicottian terms, we realise the importance of holding. When the separation occurs, the baby is left alone. The mother's representation may be suspended, and replaced by many substitutes. What is of the greatest importance is the *introjected construction of a framing structure [structure encadrante]* analogous to the mother's arms in the holding. This framing structure can tolerate the absence of representation because it holds the psychic space, like Bion's container. As long as the framing structure 'holds' the mind, the negative hallucination can be replaced by hallucinatory wish fulfilment or fantasy. But when the baby is confronted with the death experience, the frame becomes unable to create substitute representations – it holds only the void. This means the non-existence of the object or of any substitute object. The negative hallucination of the object cannot be overcome; the negative does not lead to an alternative positive substitution. Even the badness of the object and fantasised destructiveness will not do. It is the mind, that is, mental activity giving birth to representations, which is under the threat of being destroyed, in the frame. At other times it is the framing structure itself that is damaged: here we have disintegration.

Winnicott's ideas come very close to mine when we consider the pathological issues. We both agree, for instance, that as a consequence of unbearable separation, that which is usually described in terms of aggression, anger, destruction, etc. can manifest itself in a very different way. In his words, what happens is a fading of the internal representation and, in mine, a destructive negative hallucination of the object. We both think that the mechanism operating here is decathexis. When Winnicott speaks of the negative side of relationships, he means 'the gradual failure that has to be experienced by the child when the parents are not available' (1971, p. 21). This lack of availability of the parents gives rise to two different experiences. One is the feeling of the badness of the object with all the aggression included in crying, screaming, being in a state of agitation and turmoil; here the negative is identified with the bad as the opposite to the positive, namely the good. Otherwise, this unavailability is related to the non-presence of the object. You will notice that I do not use the word absence, because in the word absence there is the hope of a return of the presence. It is also not a loss because this would mean that the loss could be mourned. The reference to the negative in this second instance is to the non-existence, the void, the emptiness, in other words, the blankness. These two aspects should be differentiated. Winnicott's contribution is to show how this negative, the non-existence, will become, at some point, the only thing that is real. What happens afterwards is that even if the object reappears, the realness of the object is still related to its non-existence. The return of the presence of the object is not enough to heal the disastrous effects of its too long absence. Non-existence has taken possession of the mind, erasing the representations of the object that preceded its absence. This is an irreversible step, at least until treatment.

What is described here is constant in these cases, many of them presenting negative therapeutic reaction. In fact, in these cases neither the analyst nor the patient exist periodically in the session. These defences are mobilised each time the material comes closer to anything that is significant. The patient's mind stops registering the interpretations of the analyst. The interpretations are blotted out, the patient says his mind is blank, no associations are produced. The analytic process is paralysed for some time. The 'journey' of Freud's work could be described as starting from *neurosis as the negative of perversion to the negative therapeutic reaction*. In my mind, some aspects of these patients have not been described by Winnicott. One is struck by the fact that they seem so vulnerable, so fragile, and though they have an extreme rigidity and stubbornness, are animated by hidden feelings of revenge, which they express in an impossibility to change, or to invest new fields of experience. They seem to be bound to repetition compulsion. All this aspect of the relationship is related to what I have called *primary anality* (1993b), which is differentiated from ordinary anal eroticism because of the narcissistic aspects of the fixation. The end of my session with the patient shows her concern about the toilet. It is one of the many indications of these urethral and anal fixations to which Winnicott does not seem to have paid sufficient attention, probably because they belonged to the drives, whose role he may have underestimated, focusing his observation on the objects and the space. In fact, I believe that these aspects of the drives have to be considered together with this object relationship, each one shedding light on the other.

Winnicott developed some of the ideas I am presenting here in one of his last papers, which appears retrospectively as an important one for the understanding of his work and for his readers as well. I am referring here to 'The use of an object' (1969), in which we can witness the enormous amount of destruction implicated in the repeated annihilation of the object, where the ordinary visible features of aggression are missing. Winnicott's idea of the transitional objects and transitional phenomena has taught me something more. Speaking of objects, we should not restrict ourselves to our relationships with existing objects (whether internal or external) but we have to think also of the power of the human mind to constantly create new objects – which I call the objectualising function (1984).[8] We create objects not only from our relation with the outside world, but we supply our internal world with the infinite capacity to create objects. Freud understood this well, in his description of melancholy, where the ego itself can offer itself as a sacrifice to replace the lost object – or in identification, when, imagining their dialogue, Freud has the ego saying to the id: 'Look, you can love me too – I am so like the object' (1923, p. 30). And, finally, in sublimation we create new and non-existent objects. The objects of sublimation are not only the objects that are involved in the process of sublimation but the activity of sublimation itself. The object of the sublimation of the painter is not only the naked body of the woman, but painting itself. It is painting that which becomes our shared object beyond the representation of what is painted: the nude and its origins in the child's experience.

On the other hand, what has been called, probably improperly, death instinct, is based on a *disobjectualising function*, that is, the process by which an object loses its specific individuality, its uniqueness for us, and becomes any object, or no object at all. A raincoat fetishist does not bother about who wears the raincoat – he is only interested in the dead stuff of the raincoat. The disobjectualising function implies a (negative) decathexis of objects external, internal or even transitional. The so-called death instinct becomes an inclination to self-disappearance. It is linked less with aggression than with nothingness. Long ago, Bion made the difference between the 'no-thing' and the nothing.

Let us go back for a while to prehistoric representations. This is not speculation, like the earliest mother–baby relationship of which, in fact, we know very little. Prehistoric man designed all sorts of drawings in his caves: finger printings, representations of women with large breasts, wild animals, mammoths, rhinoceroses, lions. But on some parts of the ceiling of the caves there were other representations: what prehistorians call *negative hands*. To represent the hands, prehistoric man used two devices. The simplest was to paint the hand and to make an impression on the wall, leaving a direct trace of it. The second was more indirect and sophisticated. Here the hand that draws does not draw itself. Instead it is placed on the wall of the cave and allows the colours all around it to spread out. Then it separates from the wall, and a non-drawn hand appears. Such could be the result of the physical separation from the mother's body.

Prehistoric man did not expect us to know what the negative is about.

© The Institute of Psycho-Analysis

Notes

1   The first time I mentioned the unnoticed importance of the negative in Winnicott's work was during the discussion of a Conference of English Speaking Members of European Societies, in London in October 1976. Masud Khan, the unquestionable expert on Winnicott, replied publicly that I had misquoted Winnicott and that he never said or wrote anything of the sort. Those who knew Khan will not be surprised by such a radical but unfortunately wrong statement.

2   The paper was read at the British Psycho-Analytical Society on 30 May 1951; first publication in 1953; second publication in 1975.

3   In this last version the final lines, about psychopathology, are omitted. So is the discussion of Wulff's paper 'Fetishism and object choice in early childhood', 1946. I will come back to the significance of this self-censorship or change of mind.

4   It is this sub-section that has been published separately. Winnicott gives two references: *Child Psychology and Psychiatry*, Vol. 1 (1960) and *The Maturational Processes and the Facilitating Environment* (1965), London: Hogarth Press.

5   Winnicott is thinking here of the connection between what he says and Melanie Klein.

6   The 1951 text has been modified here, as Winnicott notes for the reader. The original mentioned the word 'badness' before the term 'failure'. Badness disap-

pears in *Playing and Reality*, probably because it is too evocative of Melanie Klein's terminology.

7 One understands here that the concept of absence has to be understood beyond its manifest meaning.

8 '*Pulsion de mort, narcissisme négatif, fonction désobjectalisante*' in Green (1984); reprinted in Green (1993a); and '*L'objet et la fonction objectalisante*', in Green (1995).

References

Abram, J. (1996) *The Language of Winnicott*. London: Karnac Books.

Freud, S. (1923) The Ego and the Id. *S.E.* 19.

Gabbard, G. O. (1997) A reconsideration of objectivity in the analyst. *International Journal of Psycho-Analysis*, 78: 15–28.

Green, A. (1975) The analyst, symbolization and absence in the analytic setting. *International Journal of Psycho-Analysis*, 56: 1–22.

—— (1984) Pulsion de mort, narcissisme négatif, fonction désobjectalisante. Reprinted in *Le Travail du négatif*. Paris: Presses Universitaires de France, pp. 49–59.

—— (1986) The dead mother. In A. Green *On Private Madness*. Original publication 'La mère morte', in *Narcissisme de vie, narcissisme de mort*. Paris: Editions Minuit, 1983, pp. 222–53.

—— (1986) *On Private Madness*, London: Hogarth Press.

—— (1993a) *Le Travail du négatif*. Paris: Editions Minuit.

—— (1993b) L'analité primaire dans la relation anale. In B. Brusset and C. Couvreur (eds) *La Névrose obsessionnelle. Monographies de la Revue Française de Psychanalyse*. Paris: Presses Universitaires de France.

—— (1995) L'objet et la fonction objectalisante. In *Propédeutique, la métapsychologie revisitée*. Paris: Editions Champvallon.

Newman, A. (1995) *Non Compliance in Winnicott's Words*. London: Free Association Books.

Ogden, T. (1994a) The analytic third: working with intersubjective clinical facts. *International Journal of Psycho-Analysis*, 75: 3–19.

—— (1994b) *Subjects of Analysis*. New York: Jason Aronson.

Winnicott, D. W. (1953a) Transitional objects and transitional phenomena. *International Journal of Psycho-Analysis*, 34: 89–96.

—— (1953b) Transitional objects and transitional phenomena. In *Playing and Reality*. London: Tavistock, pp. 1–25.

—— (1953c) Transitional objects and transitional phenomena. In *Through Paediatrics to Psycho-Analysis*. London: Hogarth Press, 1975, pp. 229–42.

—— (1960) String. *Journal of Child Psychology and Psychiatry*, 1: 229–42.

—— (1965) *The Maturational Processes and the Facilitating Environment*. London: Hogarth Press.

—— (1969) The use of an object. *International Journal of Psycho-Analysis*, 50: 711–16.

—— (1971) *Playing and Reality*. London: Tavistock.

—— (1975) *Through Paediatrics to Psycho-Analysis*. London: Hogarth Press and the Institute of Psycho-Analysis.

Wulff, E. (1946). Fetishism and object choice in early childhood. *Psychoanalytic Quarterly*, 15: 450–71.

INDEX